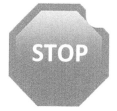

FREE BONUS CONTENT!

Did you purchase a **new** copy of this book (not used)? If so, you're eligible to receive FREE bonus content worth more than $30! You don't want to miss this! Here's how it works:

Send an email to **free@rxstudyguides.com** with "FREE BONUS" in the subject line and include the information outlined below in the body of the email.

1. Your full name and mailing address.
2. Proof of purchase (e.g., a screenshot of your receipt showing that you purchased the book in "new" condition). Please note that customers who purchased this book in "used" condition are not eligible to receive the free bonus content.

After we receive your email, we'll send your free bonus content!

Please note that the bonus content may change over time and that all bonus content is available only while supplies last.

Thank you for choosing *PTCB Exam Simplified*!

Kind regards,
David A Heckman, PharmD
Author of *PTCB Exam Simplified 4th Edition*

"Whatever you do, work heartily, as for the Lord and not for men"
- Colossians 3:23 [ESV]

"And let us not grow weary of doing good, for in due season we will reap, if we do not give up."
- Galatians 6:9 [ESV]

PTCB® EXAM
SIMPLIFIED

PHARMACY TECHNICIAN CERTIFICATION EXAM
STUDY GUIDE

4TH EDITION

BY DAVID A HECKMAN, PHARMD

PTCB® Exam Simplified: Pharmacy Technician Certification Exam Study Guide, 4th Edition

ISBN-13: 978-1942682127

Book cover design by Keeling Design & Media, Inc.

Published by David Heckman Media

Printed in the United States of America

UP TO DATE FOR THE NEW PHARMACY TECHNICIAN CERTIFICATION EXAM CONTENT OUTLINE

The Pharmacy Technician Certification Board introduced a new content outline for the Pharmacy Technician Certification Exam effective January 1st, 2020. According to the outline, exam content will now be organized into the following four knowledge areas:

1. Medications (40% of exam)
2. Federal Requirements (12.5% of exam)
3. Patient Safety & Quality Assurance (26.25% of exam)
4. Order Entry and Processing (21.25% of exam)

Guided by the updated exam content outline, PTCB Exam Simplified (4rd Edition) provides a thorough review of the most important information relevant to these four knowledge areas.

YOU MUST READ THIS CAREFULLY!

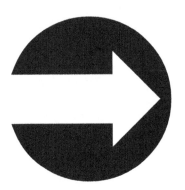

DO THESE THREE THINGS, AND PASS THE EXAM
<u>GUARANTEED</u>!

I get it! You don't have a lot of time to spend preparing for this exam. You need to cut to the chase and get to the point where you can pass! Here's how to do it in <u>three simple steps</u>:

1. Study the content outlined on the PTCB exam blueprint

    I created *PTCB Exam Simplified 4th Edition* over a multi-year period specifically to cover everything on the current PTCB exam blueprint. There's no fluff. Nothing from the old blueprints. Just the new stuff. Nothing to throw you off-track.

2. Memorize the basics

    To help you do this, I created the proprietary *PTCB Exam Cheat Sheet*. In the past, I sold this cheat sheet for $10+, but now I'm giving it away for **FREE** to anyone who buys a new copy of *PTCB Exam Simplified 4th Edition* (not available for customers who purchase the book used). I will need your mailing address and proof of purchase so I can send it to you. It's easy, just follow the instructions on page 1.

3. Practice, practice, practice

    Do my practice exams! I included one practice exam in the book and there's a second practice exam I posted for FREE at cphtacademy.com. But that's not all! I have a package of two more practice exams which I normally sell for $24.99 at cphtacademy.com, but anyone who buys this book new can access those exams for **FREE** (not available for customers who purchase the book used). As with the cheat sheet, just follow the instructions on page 1 to claim your free bonus content.

Thoroughly complete each of the three steps outlined above, and you will pass the exam, <u>I guarantee it</u> (continue reading)! *PTCB Exam Simplified 4th Edition* costs about $20 more than the average competitor's study guide. Why? More value! I'm so confident that you'll pass the certification exam using this book (along with the $30+ worth of bonus content) that I'm going to put my money where my mouth is! If you purchase a brand-new copy of *PTCB Exam Simplified 4th Edition* and use it with the free bonus content, then still fail the exam, you can notify me via email according to the instructions on page 241. I'll issue a $20 credit in the form of an Amazon gift card. How can I be so confident that this book (and the bonus content) will help you achieve a passing score? Because I sent a survey to more than 1,000 people preparing for the PTCB exam and among respondents who said they used my book, the pass rate was outstanding–significantly higher than the average PTCB-reported pass rate.

All the best,
David A Heckman, PharmD
Author of *PTCB Exam Simplified*

P.S. I know you can (and will) pass the exam!

TABLE OF CONTENTS

TABLE OF CONTENTS

ABOUT THE PTCB EXAM

- $129 exam registration fee.
- Administered at Pearson VUE testing centers.
- Computer-based exam.
- 90 multiple-choice questions.
- Basic calculator provided.
- No penalties for guessing.
- 120 minutes to complete.
    - 5-minute introductory tutorial.
    - 110-minute examination.
    - 5-minute exit survey.
- Scaled scores range from 1000 – 1600.
    - Must achieve a scaled score of 1400 or higher to pass.

A QUICK NOTE
BEFORE YOU GET STARTED

To present information in an order consistent with the PTCB exam content outline, the section on medical terminology is located toward the end of this study guide (on pages 192–200). However, you may gain the most benefit by reviewing this section first.

KNOWLEDGE AREA #1
MEDICATIONS

REVIEWING MEDICATIONS BY DRUG CLASS

Drugs are grouped into categories–referred to as "drug classes"–based on their pharmacology. Drugs in the same drug class share the same pharmacologic mechanism of action. Studying the pharmacology of one drug at a time is tedious and inefficient. To simplify and expedite the process, we will present medications one drug class at a time. Assume that the drugs discussed in this section are prescription-only ("Rx only") unless specified otherwise. Topics covered will include uses (indications), mechanisms of action (pharmacology), side effects, common drug interactions, and other noteworthy details.

UNDERSTANDING HIGH BLOOD PRESSURE

High blood pressure (hypertension) is a chronic medical condition. Over many years, the force of high pressure inside the blood vessels causes damage, which creates rough patches. Cholesterol tends to stick to and build up on these rough patches, forming little mounds. We call this process atherosclerosis, and it impedes the flow of blood through the blood vessel, which can cause problems such as coronary artery disease, angina, and myocardial infarction. Hypertension is quite common, and several drugs are available to treat it.

INTRODUCTION TO ACE INHIBITORS AND ARBs

WHAT ARE ACE INHIBITORS AND ARBs?

ACE inhibitor is an abbreviation for angiotensin converting enzyme inhibitor. ARB is an abbreviation for Angiotensin Receptor Blocker. These two drug classes are very similar; both work by reducing the effect of a hormone called angiotensin, a potent vasoconstrictor that raises blood pressure. The enzyme abbreviated as "ACE" converts angiotensin to an even more powerful blood vessel constricting hormone called angiotensin II, but the story doesn't end there. Angiotensin II goes on to stimulate the release of another hormone called aldosterone, which causes salt retention, further increasing blood pressure. By interfering with angiotensin before it becomes angiotensin II, we prevent a lot of the blood vessel constriction and salt retention that can contribute to high blood pressure. I know, it gets a little complicated, but do not be overwhelmed by all of these details. The take-home message is that ACE inhibitors and ARBs share a similar mechanism of action, and the drugs in both classes are used to reduce blood pressure in patients with hypertension.

ACE INHIBITOR vs ARB: COMPARISON OF SIDE EFFECTS

Because ACE inhibitors and ARBs share a similar mechanism of action, they also have similar side effects. Nonetheless, there are minor differences. Observe the chart below for a comparison of the most common and severe potential side effects.

Side Effect	ACE Inhibitors	ARBs
Nonproductive Cough	✓	
Hypotension	✓	✓
Hyperkalemia	✓	✓
Anaphylaxis	✓	✓

ACE INHIBITORS AND ARBs ARE BOTH PREGNANCY CATEGORY X
NEVER TO BE USED DURING PREGNANCY

ANGIOTENSIN CONVERTING ENZYME (ACE) INHIBITORS FOR HYPERTENSION

BRAND NAME	GENERIC NAME
Lotensin®	Benazepril
Vasotec®	Enalapril
Prinivil®, Zestril®	Lisinopril
Accupril®	Quinapril
Altace®	Ramipril

Note: notice the generic names of the ACE inhibitors end in "–pril."

ACE INHIBITOR DRUG NAME STEM
-PRIL

BACKGROUND
Angiotensin is a hormone produced by the kidneys that causes vasoconstriction and salt retention, both of which contribute to high blood pressure.

PHARMACOLOGY
ACE inhibitors reduce the effect of angiotensin, ultimately relaxing the blood vessels, preventing salt retention, and lowering blood pressure.

INDICATIONS
Hypertension, Heart Failure, Myocardial Infarction (Heart Attack), Kidney Protection in Diabetic Patients

SIDE EFFECTS
Nonproductive Cough, Hypotension, Hyperkalemia, Anaphylaxis (rare)

DRUG INTERACTIONS
ACE inhibitors can cause high potassium (hyperkalemia), which can lead to life-threatening cardiac arrhythmias. Patients using potassium supplements or potassium-sparing diuretics are more likely to experience hyperkalemia while taking ACE inhibitors.

NOTES
ACE inhibitors are known to cause birth defects when taken during pregnancy. They should never be used during pregnancy (pregnancy category X). About 20% of patients on ACE inhibitors experience a dry, nonproductive cough. The only way to eliminate this side effect is to discontinue the ACE inhibitor. Many prescribers solve this problem by switching to an ARB, which produces the same pharmacologic effect without the potential to cause a dry cough.

```
DO NOT USE IF
PREGNANT
```

A COMMON SIDE EFFECT OF ALL BLOOD PRESSURE-LOWERING DRUGS

All blood pressure-lowering drugs have the potential to cause hypotension (abnormally low blood pressure), particularly when taken at doses that exceed what was prescribed or when exposed to other conditions such as dehydration. The patient should periodically monitor their blood pressure to ensure their blood pressure is under control. For most patients, the target blood pressure is < 130/80 mmHg; however, if a patient is experiencing symptoms of hypotension and their blood pressure reading is lower than 90/60 mmHg, then they should seek medical attention for hypotension.

ANGIOTENSIN RECEPTOR BLOCKERS (ARBs)
FOR HYPERTENSION

BRAND NAME	GENERIC NAME
Edarbi®	Azilsartan
Atacand®	Candesartan
Avapro®	Irbesartan
Cozaar®	Losartan
Benicar®	Olmesartan
Micardis®	Telmisartan
Diovan®	Valsartan

Note: notice how the generic names of the ARBs all end in "–sartan."

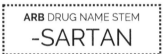

ARB DRUG NAME STEM
-SARTAN

BACKGROUND
For angiotensin to exert its effect (blood vessel constriction), it must bind to angiotensin receptors.

PHARMACOLOGY
ARBs reduce the effect of angiotensin by preventing angiotensin receptor binding. Ultimately, this relaxes the blood vessels, reduces salt retention, and lowers blood pressure.

INDICATIONS
Hypertension, Heart Failure, Myocardial Infarction (Heart Attack) Stroke Prevention, Renal Protection in Diabetic Patients

SIDE EFFECTS
Fatigue, Dizziness, Hyperkalemia, Hypotension, Anaphylaxis (rare).

DRUG INTERACTIONS
Since ARBs can increase the level of potassium in the blood, concurrent use of potassium supplements and potassium-sparing diuretics will increase the risk of hyperkalemia.

NOTES
As with the ACE inhibitors, ARBs can cause birth defects when used during pregnancy. They should never be used during pregnancy (pregnancy category X).

DO NOT USE IF
PREGNANT

INTRODUCTION TO DIURETICS

WHAT EXACTLY IS URINE?

The kidneys work as filters for circulating blood. As the heart pumps blood back and forth through arteries and veins, the kidneys continuously function to remove waste products from the blood, producing urine. Everything that ends up in the urine was once a part of the blood. This includes water, electrolytes, metabolized vitamins, and even medications.

HOW KIDNEYS MANAGE THE BALANCE OF ELECTROLYTES

Nutrients and water from food and beverages pass from the intestinal tract into the bloodstream through a process called "absorption." Nutrients include fat, protein, carbohydrates, vitamins, and electrolytes (e.g., sodium, potassium, calcium, magnesium). Electrolytes are needed mainly for nerve and muscle function. If electrolyte levels are too low or too high, the consequences can be severe, including seizures, cardiac arrhythmias, and even death. The kidneys continuously work to maintain the proper balance of electrolytes. They accomplish this by diverting electrolytes from the blood into the urine when the concentration in the blood is high and preventing electrolytes from entering the urine when the concentration is low.

THE RELATIONSHIP BETWEEN SODIUM AND BLOOD PRESSURE

By a process called osmosis, sodium attracts water. Excess salt (sodium chloride) in the bloodstream causes water retention, which increases blood pressure.

DIURETICS AND SODIUM

Diuretics increase urine production by forcing the kidneys to divert more sodium from the blood into the urine. By osmosis, water follows sodium into the urine. When water leaves the bloodstream, the blood becomes more concentrated and takes up less space in the blood vessels. Ultimately, this causes blood pressure to decrease.

DIURETICS AND POTASSIUM

There are three classes of diuretics: 1) Thiazide diuretics, 2) Loop diuretics, and 3) Potassium-sparing diuretics. Diuretics divert sodium from the blood into the urine, but in doing so, they also divert potassium from the blood into the urine. This is a side effect, and it may cause an abnormally low level of potassium in the blood. Potassium-sparing diuretics are the exception. They divert sodium into the urine without causing a loss of potassium; however, they tend to have a weaker blood pressure-lowering effect when compared to the other types of diuretics.

THIAZIDE DIURETICS FOR HYPERTENSION

BRAND NAME	GENERIC NAME
Hygroton®, Thalitone®	Chlorthalidone
Microzide®	Hydrochlorothiazide

BACKGROUND
Sodium, found in salt, is associated with water retention and, consequently, hypertension.

PHARMACOLOGY
Thiazide diuretics increase the transfer of salt and water from the blood to urine, thus reducing blood pressure.

INDICATIONS
Hypertension, Edema

SIDE EFFECTS
Hypotension, Hypokalemia, Hyperuricemia, Muscle Cramps (caused by low potassium), Cardiac Arrhythmias (also caused by low potassium), Photosensitivity (predisposition to sunburn), SJS (rare)

DRUG INTERACTIONS
Potential for severe hypotension when combined with other blood pressure-lowering drugs (ACE inhibitors, ARBs, loop diuretics, etc.). Also, potential for severe hypokalemia when used with loop diuretics.

NOTES
Thiazides share a similarity with sulfonamide antibiotics, not in their mechanism of action, but their chemical structure. Because of this similarity, patients with a sulfa allergy may also be allergic to thiazide diuretics.

POTASSIUM REPLACEMENT WITH THIAZIDE AND LOOP DIURETICS

As we have discussed, thiazide diuretics and loop diuretics deplete potassium. For this reason, many prescribers will take measures to prevent hypokalemia in patients receiving one or both of these diuretics. Expect to see one or more of the following strategies:

1. The prescriber instructs the patient to "take with a banana or orange juice."
2. The prescriber issues a potassium supplement (K-Dur®, Klor-Con®).
3. The prescriber issues a combination drug product (discussed below).

Note: Bananas and orange juice are naturally high in potassium.

HYDROCHLOROTHIAZIDE COMBINATION PRODUCTS

Manufacturers produce several thiazide-ARB and thiazide-ACE inhibitor combinations for a couple of reasons: #1 Most patients require more than one hypertension drug to achieve their blood pressure goal, and #2 ARBs and ACE inhibitors can oppose the potassium-depleting effect of thiazide diuretics. See the two most popular combinations below.

BRAND NAME	GENERIC NAME
Zestoretic®	Lisinopril/Hydrochlorothiazide
Hyzaar®	Losartan/Hydrochlorothiazide

LOOP DIURETICS FOR HYPERTENSION

BRAND NAME	GENERIC NAME
Bumex®	Bumetanide
Edecrin®	Ethacrynic Acid
Lasix®	Furosemide
Demadex®	Torsemide

BACKGROUND
Sodium, a major component of table salt (NaCl), promotes water retention and, consequently, hypertension.

PHARMACOLOGY
Similar to thiazide diuretics, loop diuretics promote the transfer of salt and water from the blood to the urine, thus reducing blood pressure.

INDICATIONS
Hypertension, Edema

SIDE EFFECTS
Hypokalemia, Hypotension, Muscle Cramps (caused by low potassium), Cardiac Arrhythmias (caused by low potassium), Photosensitivity (predisposition to sunburn), SJS (rare)

DRUG INTERACTIONS
Virtually the same drug interactions as with the thiazide diuretics – additive hypotension when combined with other drugs that lower blood pressure, and additive hypokalemia when used with thiazide diuretics.

NOTES
Loop diuretics are the most effective type of diuretic available. They have the potential to cause life-threatening potassium depletion if misused.

MNEMONIC FOR REMEMBERING THE LOOP DIURETIC GENERIC NAMES

"BEAU-TI-FUL"

When we breakdown the word "beautiful" into its three syllables (beau-ti-ful), we see that each syllable begins with a letter corresponding to the first letter of the generic name of the most commonly used loop diuretics (bumetanide, torsemide, and furosemide).

The "B" in **Beau-** corresponds to the "B" in **Bumetanide**.
The "T" in **-Ti-** corresponds to the "T" in **Torsemide**.
The "F" in **–Ful** corresponds to the "F" in **Furosemide**.

EXPECT TO SEE UNIQUE INSTRUCTIONS FROM TIME TO TIME

Since prescribers may issue loop diuretics to treat edema in patients with heart failure, we occasionally see odd-looking instructions. For instance, "take one tablet by mouth once daily if weight increases > 2 pounds in 24 hours." Why? Rapid weight gain is usually a sign of fluid retention ("water weight"), which can cause severe problems in patients with heart failure.

POTASSIUM-SPARING DIURETICS
FOR HYPERTENSION

BRAND NAME	GENERIC NAME
Midamor®	Amiloride
Inspra®	Eplerenone
Aldactone®	Spironolactone
Dyrenium®	Triamterene

BACKGROUND
Hypokalemia is a common side effect caused by diuretics.

PHARMACOLOGY
Increase the amount of salt and water that leaves the body via the urine, but without causing low potassium.

INDICATIONS
Hypertension, Heart Failure

SIDE EFFECTS
Hyperkalemia, Hypotension

DRUG INTERACTIONS
Because they work in a way that prevents potassium loss, potassium-sparing diuretics may cause high potassium levels in the blood (hyperkalemia). The combined use of potassium supplements increases this risk.

NOTES
Potassium-sparing diuretics have a mechanism that does not work quite as well as the thiazide or loop diuretics (see illustration below), but, as the name suggests, their use does not cause a reduction in blood potassium levels. Rather, they may elevate blood potassium. For this reason, when patients need more than one medication to achieve their blood pressure goal, one option prescribers may use is to combine a potassium-sparing diuretic with a thiazide diuretic. This combination induces diuresis and lowers blood pressure by two different mechanisms, and, since they have opposing effects on potassium levels, it helps prevent potassium imbalances as well. Note the combination drugs below.

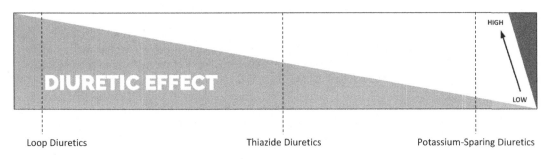

Loop Diuretics   Thiazide Diuretics   Potassium-Sparing Diuretics

POTASSIUM-SPARING + THIAZIDE DIURETIC COMBINATION DRUGS

BRAND NAME	GENERIC NAME
Aldactazide®	Spironolactone/Hydrochlorothiazide
Dyazide®, Maxzide®	Triamterene/Hydrochlorothiazide

INTRODUCTION TO ALPHA AND BETA RECEPTORS

BLOOD VESSELS HAVE MUSCLE

The cardiovascular system is composed of the heart and blood vessels. The blood vessels provide a structural, tube-like network to channel blood to and from every living part of the body, and the heart provides the force needed to circulate the blood through the vessels. You may already know that the heart is a muscle, but did you know that blood vessels are lined with muscle tissue as well? The muscle in blood vessels will constrict to limit blood flow and relax to increase blood flow. For example, when you are engaged in vigorous physical activity, the blood vessels carrying blood to the intestines will contract, while the blood vessels that carry blood to the skeletal muscles will expand. Why is this important? Because of the effect on blood pressure. Blood vessel constriction increases blood pressure, and blood vessel relaxation decreases blood pressure. Furthermore, we can control these processes pharmacologically.

ALPHA AND BETA RECEPTORS

Alpha and beta receptors are involved in regulating the cardiovascular system (the heart and blood vessels). Alpha$_1$ and alpha$_2$ receptors regulate blood pressure via constriction and relaxation of blood vessels. Beta-receptors regulate chronotropy/inotropy (i.e., the and force of the heartbeat), which also affects blood pressure, and airway dilation/constriction.

ALPHA$_1$ RECEPTOR ACTIVATION
↑ BLOOD PRESSURE

Activation of alpha$_1$ receptors by adrenaline and norepinephrine causes blood vessel constriction, which raises blood pressure.

ALPHA$_2$ RECEPTOR ACTIVATION
↓ BLOOD PRESSURE

Activation of alpha$_2$ receptors reduces the amount of adrenaline and norepinephrine in the blood, which ultimately reduces blood pressure.

BETA RECEPTOR ACTIVATION
↑ HEART RATE & BLOOD PRESSURE

Activation of beta-receptors causes the heart to beat faster and harder, which raises blood pressure. Activation of beta-receptors also causes the airways to open up. Blocking beta-receptors causes the heart to relax and has a blood pressure-lowering effect. Certain beta-receptor blockers may cause breathing problems for patients with asthma or COPD.

ALPHA₁ RECEPTOR ANTAGONISTS (ALPHA₁ BLOCKERS)
FOR HYPERTENSION

BRAND NAME	GENERIC NAME
Uroxatral®	Afluzosin
Cardura®	Doxazosin
Rapaflo®	Silodosin
Flomax®	Tamsulosin
Hytrin®	Terazosin

Note: notice how the generic names of the aplha₁-blockers all end in "–osin."

BACKGROUND
Activation of alpha₁ receptors causes blood vessels to constrict.

> ALPHA1 BLOCKER DRUG NAME STEM
> ## -OSIN

PHARMACOLOGY
Prevent the activation of alpha₁ receptors, leading to the relaxation of blood vessels. These drugs also happen to relax muscles in the bladder neck and prostate, which is why medications from this class are also used to treat enlarged prostate (benign prostatic hyperplasia).

INDICATIONS
Hypertension, Benign Prostatic Hyperplasia (BPH)

SIDE EFFECTS
Orthostatic Hypotension (blood pressure drops quickly upon changing from the sitting position to standing), Dizziness, Syncope

DRUG INTERACTIONS
Increased risk of hypotension when used with other blood pressure-lowering drugs.

NOTES
BPH is a condition in which the prostate gland is larger than normal. The main symptom is the obstruction of urinary outflow. There are alpha₁ receptors in the prostate and the neck of the bladder, which is located next to the prostate. By blocking alpha₁ receptors, the muscles in the prostate gland and bladder neck relax, allowing urine to flow out unobstructed. Alpha₁ blockers also relax blood vessels at other locations throughout the body. Consequently, some alpha1 blockers are designed to target BPH, while others target high blood pressure.

EMERGENCY ANAPHYLAXIS

People with a severe allergy, such as to bee stings, often carry an EpiPen®, an auto-injector device containing epinephrine (adrenaline). Patients inject the contents of the EpiPen® into their thigh in the event of anaphylaxis. During anaphylaxis, patients typically have dangerously low blood pressure and severe difficulty breathing. The active ingredient in the EpiPen®, epinephrine, stimulates both alpha and beta receptors, leading to blood vessel constriction, stronger and faster heartbeats, and dilation of the airways. While EpiPen is the most popular device of its kind, other brands exist (see below).

BRAND NAME	GENERIC NAME
Auvi-Q®	Epinephrine
Symjepi™	Epinephrine

ALPHA₂ RECEPTOR AGONISTS (ALPHA₂ AGONISTS)
FOR HYPERTENSION

BRAND NAME	GENERIC NAME
Catapress®, Kapvay®	Clonidine
Intuniv®, Tenex®	Guanfacine
Aldomet®	Methyldopa

BACKGROUND
The nervous system releases norepinephrine all the time. More in times of stress, less in times of rest, but some level of norepinephrine is always present. Our nerve cells have regulators known as alpha₂ receptors, which prevent too much norepinephrine from releasing at one time. Consider this analogy: A thermostat is to heat from a furnace as alpha₂ receptors are to norepinephrine from the nervous system. When the temperature in a room gets too high, the thermostat signals the furnace to stop releasing heat. Likewise, when the norepinephrine level reaches a certain point in the bloodstream, alpha₂ receptors signal the nervous system to stop (or reduce) the release of norepinephrine.

PHARMACOLOGY
Activate aplha₂ receptors, which decreases norepinephrine levels and, consequently, lowers blood pressure.

INDICATIONS
Hypertension, ADHD

SIDE EFFECTS
Bradycardia, Hypotension, Drowsiness, Rebound Hypertension

DRUG INTERACTIONS
Increased risk of hypotension when used with other drugs that decrease blood pressure. Increased risk of bradycardia when used with drugs that decrease heart rate (e.g., beta-blockers).

PATIENTS SHOULD NOT DISCONTINUE ABRUPTLY
DUE TO RISK OF REBOUND HYPERTENSION AND WITHDRAWAL SYMPTOMS
Rebound hypertension and withdrawal symptoms, including tachycardia, tremor, nervousness, agitation, and sweating, can occur with abrupt discontinuation of an alpha₂ agonist, particularly when used for ≥ 2 months. To discontinue, follow the advice of a physician and reduce the dose gradually over several days.

ALDOMET® (METHYLDOPA)
THE DRUG OF CHOICE FOR HYPERTENSION DURING PREGNANCY
Methyldopa is relatively safe and effective during pregnancy. Most pregnant women take prenatal vitamins that contain iron, which may reduce the absorption and effect of methyldopa. This drug-vitamin interaction can be avoided by separating the administration of iron by at least two hours.

BETA RECEPTOR ANTAGONISTS (BETA-BLOCKERS)
FOR HYPERTENSION

BRAND NAME	GENERIC NAME
Sectral®	Acebutalol
Tenormin®	Atenolol
Coreg®	Carvedilol
Trandate®	Labetalol
Toprol XL®	Metoprolol succinate (extended release)
Lopressor®	Metoprolol tartrate (immediate release)
Inderal®	Propranolol
Betapace®	Sotalol

Note: notice how the generic names of most of the beta-blockers end in "–olol."

BACKGROUND
Beta-receptor activation increases the heart rate, increases the force of the heartbeat, and dilates the airways in the lungs.

BETA BLOCKER DRUG NAME STEM
-OLOL

PHARMACOLOGY
Prevent the activation of beta-receptors, reducing the heart rate, and reducing the force of the heartbeat. Beta-blockers also relax the blood vessels. These effects lead to decreased blood pressure and heart rate.

INDICATIONS
Hypertension, Angina, Atrial Fibrillation, Myocardial Infarction, Migraine Prevention

SIDE EFFECTS
Bradycardia, Exacerbation of Asthma or COPD, Hypotension, Fatigue

DRUG INTERACTIONS
Certain beta-blockers can interfere with the effect of some asthma medications, like albuterol, that work by activating beta-receptors. The risk of hypotension increases when combined with other drugs that lower blood pressure.

NOTES
Abrupt cessation of a beta-blocker can cause severe withdrawal symptoms. If a patient suddenly stops taking a beta-blocker, they can have a heart attack. If a patient mentions anything about deciding to stop taking a medication, alert the pharmacist.

THE MANY USES OF BETA BLOCKERS
As you can see from the long and diverse list of indications, beta-blockers are versatile. They can treat a variety of conditions, mostly heart-related. I want to take a second to explain why. Since beta-blockers decrease the rate and force of the heartbeat, they reduce stress on the heart. The heart does not have to work as hard. As a result, the heart requires less oxygen. Remember, the whole issue with angina and heart attacks is that the heart is not receiving enough oxygen. Beta-blockers also relax blood vessels, which is perfect for improving blood flow to an oxygen-deprived heart. Atrial fibrillation is another condition where a beta-blocker can be beneficial. Atrial fibrillation is a type of cardiac arrhythmia – the rhythm of the heartbeat is abnormal. One way to normalize the rhythm is to slow down the heart using a beta-blocker.

WARNING FOR PATIENTS WITH DIABETES
Beta-blockers can mask several signs of hypoglycemia, including tachycardia and tremors.
Sweating is one of the few signs of hypoglycemia that is not masked by a beta-blocker.

CALCIUM CHANNEL BLOCKERS (CCBs)
FOR HYPERTENSION

BRAND NAME	GENERIC NAME
Norvasc®	Amlodipine
Cardizem®, Tiazac®, Taztia XT®	Diltiazem
Plendil®	Felodipine
Cardene®	Nicardipine
Procardia®	Nifedipine
Sular®	Nisoldipine
Isoptin®, Verelan®, Calan®	Verapamil

BACKGROUND
The muscle tissue that forms the heart and lines the blood vessels uses calcium for effective contraction.

PHARMACOLOGY
Reduce the amount of calcium available to cardiac and vascular muscle cells. With less calcium, the heart beats with less force, and the blood vessels relax, both leading to a decrease in blood pressure.

INDICATIONS
Hypertension, Angina

SIDE EFFECTS
Headache, Fatigue, Edema

DRUG INTERACTIONS
The risk of hypotension increases when taken with other drugs that lower blood pressure.

Note: "Angina" is chest pain resulting from inadequate blood flow to the heart.

THE #1 SIDE EFFECT: HEADACHE
Some prominent side effects of calcium channel blockers (e.g., edema) are caused by vasodilation. The most common side effect is a headache, which occurs when dilated blood vessels in the head can press on nearby pain receptors (nociceptors).

PATIENTS SHOULD AVOID GRAPEFRUIT JUICE
Grapefruit juice contains compounds that inhibit a key metabolic enzyme involved in the elimination of many calcium channel blockers. Consequently, it is prudent for patients to avoid the consumption of grapefruit or grapefruit juice while taking a calcium channel blocker.

UNDERSTANDING HIGH CHOLESTEROL

Similar to hypertension, high cholesterol is a chronic condition. Cholesterol levels must be high for several years before an adverse effect is recognized. The long-term negative impact can include coronary artery disease, angina, and myocardial infarction.

THE TWO SOURCES OF CHOLESTEROL

When we think of cholesterol, we often think of fatty food, but cholesterol actually comes from another place as well: the liver! Our livers produce cholesterol to ensure that cholesterol is present even if we are not obtaining it from food. While cholesterol can have adverse effects when levels are high, the body needs some cholesterol for essential processes like hormone production and cell wall synthesis. The amount of cholesterol produced by the liver varies from person to person, depending on genetics.

HMG-CoA REDUCTASE INHIBITORS (STATINS)
FOR HIGH CHOLESTEROL

BRAND NAME	GENERIC NAME
Lipitor®	Atorvastatin
Lescol®	Fluvastatin
Mevacor®	Lovastatin
Livalo®	Pitavastatin
Pravachol®	Pravastatin
Crestor®	Rosuvastatin
Zocor®	Simvastatin

Note: notice how the generic names end in "–statin."

STATIN DRUG NAME STEM

-STATIN

BACKGROUND
Cholesterol comes from two sources: dietary intake (food) and production by the liver.

PHARMACOLOGY
Inhibit the enzyme HMG-CoA reductase, which is the key enzyme used by the liver to produce cholesterol.

INDICATION
High Cholesterol

SIDE EFFECTS
Muscle Aches/Myopathy, Liver Damage

DRUG INTERACTIONS
Grapefruit juice, in large amounts, can interfere with the metabolism and elimination of statins, which can cause statins to accumulate in the body, eventually leading to serious health problems.

NOTES
Statins cause birth defects and should never be used during pregnancy (pregnancy category X). The liver ramps up cholesterol production at night, so statins are generally more effective when administered at night. Certain statins (e.g., atorvastatin and rosuvastatin) are eliminated from the body at a very slow rate. For this reason, it is not necessary to take atorvastatin or rosuvastatin at night; they can be taken at any time of the day. Since HMG-CoA reductase inhibitors only reduce cholesterol production and do not have an effect on dietary intake, patients should make dietary changes to reduce the amount of cholesterol they consume. How? Read nutrition labels. Avoid foods high in saturated fat and cholesterol (e.g., doughnuts, Big Macs, fried chicken).

PATIENTS SHOULD AVOID GRAPEFRUIT JUICE
Grapefruit juice contains compounds that inhibit a key metabolic enzyme involved in the elimination of many statins. Consequently, it is prudent for patients to avoid grapefruit juice while taking statins.

ALL STATINS ARE PREGNANCY CATEGORY X
Babies need cholesterol for healthy development, so statins should never be used by women who are pregnant or nursing.

DO NOT USE IF
PREGNANT OR NURSING

BILE ACID SEQUESTRANTS
FOR HIGH CHOLESTEROL

BRAND NAME	GENERIC NAME
Colestid®	Colestipol
Questran®	Cholestyramine
Welchol®	Colesevelam

BACKGROUND

The cholesterol produced by the liver becomes bile acid, a thick fluid that enters the intestinal tract and aids in the absorption of fat. Typically, the body reabsorbs/reuses bile acid are from the gastrointestinal tract.

PHARMACOLOGY

Bind to ("sequester") cholesterol from bile acid, carrying the cholesterol out of the body during defecation, which prevents cholesterol produced by the liver from being reabsorbed/reused. The liver compensates for this loss of bile acid by using cholesterol to produce more bile acid. Ultimately, this lowers cholesterol.

INDICATIONS

High Cholesterol

SIDE EFFECTS

Constipation, Flatulence

DRUG INTERACTIONS

Since bile acid sequestrants work by binding to and preventing the absorption of cholesterol from the intestinal tract, it's not surprising to learn that this class of drugs also interferes with the absorption of many medications. There are too many drug interactions to list. Generally, patients should separate the dosing of other medications by a few hours to avoid drug interactions.

VITAMIN DEFICIENCIES

Bile acids aid in the digestion of fats and fat-soluble vitamins. Since bile acid sequestrants remove bile acid form the gastrointestinal tract, fat-soluble vitamin deficiencies (A, D, E, and K) can occur, particularly with the long-term use of bile acid sequestrants.

PRESCRIBED OFF-LABEL FOR DIARRHEA

Bile acid sequestrants are so notorious for causing constipation (a side effect) that some doctors prescribe bile acid sequestrants off-label for the treatment of diarrhea.

SIMILARITIES WITH ZETIA®

Zetia® (ezetimibe) is a popular cholesterol-lowering drug that works in a way similar to bile acid sequestrants; however, ezetimibe belongs to a drug class of its own. It is a "cholesterol absorption inhibitor," and, rather than binding bile acid, it works by blocking the absorption of intestinal cholesterol from all sources (cholesterol from dietary sources and bile acid). The general concept is similar. Both drug classes reduce the amount of cholesterol that enters the bloodstream.

UNDERSTANDING BLOOD CLOTS

You bleed after cutting or scraping your skin, but after a few minutes, the blood hardens, and the bleeding stops. This is an example of blood clotting. Blood can also clot inside a blood vessel, and when it does, the results can be dangerous. A blood clot in the leg, called Deep Vein Thrombosis (DVT), can travel to the lungs and cause a potentially fatal event called a Pulmonary Embolism (PE). A blood clot in the heart can cause a Myocardial Infarction (MI), also known as a heart attack. A blood clot that travels to the brain can cause a stroke. Naturally, you're probably wondering, what exactly is a blood clot?

WHAT IS A BLOOD CLOT?

A blood clot is a clump of hard, sticky material composed of two substances – fibrin and platelets. A damaged blood vessel interacts with blood to form fibrin and to attract platelets to the site of damage. The damage can occur from a physical cut, in which case the clot forms outside of the vessel, typically on the surface of the skin. On the other hand, certain internal processes such as high blood pressure and high cholesterol can cause damage, in which case the clot forms inside the blood vessel.

PLATELETS

Platelets are a normal part of the blood. They circulate back and forth through the bloodstream, along with everything else in the blood. When a blood vessel is torn, it releases chemicals that cause platelets to gather around the damaged area and form a plug. Then fibrin comes in and reinforces the platelet plug.

FIBRIN

Fibrin forms out of a series of chemical reactions. The reactants are liquid, and like platelets, they are a normal part of the blood. On a microscopic level, fibrin resembles little strands of fiber that form a mesh-like network around the damaged area where platelets have gathered.

THE KEY TO BLOOD CLOT PREVENTION

We can prevent blood clot formation by interfering with platelet aggregation and fibrin formation. Antiplatelet drugs prevent blood clot formation by interfering with platelet aggregation. Anticoagulants, on the other hand, interfere with fibrin formation.

INCREASED BLEEDING RISK

Our goal with anticoagulant and antiplatelet therapy is to prevent blood from clotting inside the blood vessels, but in doing so, we also interfere with external blood clotting – the type of blood clotting that stops bleeding from cuts, scrapes, and bruises.

ANTICOAGULANTS FOR BLOOD CLOTS

BRAND NAME	GENERIC NAME
---	Heparin
Arixtra®	Fondaparinux
Coumadin®, Jantoven®	Warfarin
Eliquis®	Apixaban
Lovenox®	Enoxaparin
Pradaxa®	Dabigatran
Xarelto®	Rivaroxaban

BACKGROUND
Fibrin is one of the two major components of a blood clot. It forms out of a series of chemical reactions between blood and the chemicals released by a damaged blood vessel.

PHARMACOLOGY
Block/interfere with chemical reactions that lead to the formation of fibrin.

INDICATIONS
Prevention or Treatment of Blood Clots (e.g., Myocardial Infarction, Pulmonary Embolism, Venous Thromboembolism)

SIDE EFFECTS
Excessive Bleeding, Easy Bruising

DRUG INTERACTIONS
Foods, beverages, and supplements rich in vitamin K will interfere with the effect of warfarin. In addition, anticoagulants increase the risk of gastrointestinal bleeding when used with NSAIDs and aspirin.

BE ALERT FOR OTC NSAID AND ASPIRIN USE
Many people use an NSAID or aspirin over the counter for self-treatment of minor aches and pains; however, combining an NSAID or aspirin with an anticoagulant can lead to dangerous problems with bleeding, especially gastrointestinal bleeding. If you notice a patient on anticoagulant therapy approaches the pharmacy counter to purchase an NSAID or aspirin, please alert the pharmacist.

WARFARIN IS PREGNANCY CATEGORY X
NEVER TO BE USED DURING PREGNANCY

THE #1 SIDE EFFECT: BLEEDING
Bleeding associated with anticoagulant use can range from minor bleeding to life-threatening hemorrhage. Consequently, anticoagulants should not be used in patients with active pathological bleeding. Patients should report unusual bruising or bleeding to their healthcare provider.

STRESS THE IMPORTANCE OF TAKING EXACTLY AS PRESCRIBED
Compliance is important with all medications; however, the consequence of failing to take an anticoagulant as prescribed could be fatal. An overdose could cause a life-threatening hemorrhage, while missed doses could lead to a major event such as a heart attack or stroke.

ANTIPLATELETS FOR BLOOD CLOTS

BRAND NAME	GENERIC NAME
Aggrenox®	Aspirin/Dipyridamole
Bayer Aspirin®, Ecotrin®	Aspirin
Effient®	Prasugrel
Integrilin®	Eptifibatide
Plavix®	Clopidogrel
Pletal®	Cilostazol
Reopro®	Abciximab

BACKGROUND
Platelets are one of two key components of a blood clot. They aggregate around damaged blood vessels and form a plug.

PHARMACOLOGY
Prevent/interfere with platelet aggregation.

INDICATIONS
Prevention or Treatment of Blood Clots (e.g., Myocardial Infarction, Pulmonary Embolism, Venous Thromboembolism)

SIDE EFFECTS
Excessive Bleeding, Easy Bruising

DRUG INTERACTIONS
Antiplatelet drugs increase the risk of gastrointestinal bleeding when used with NSAIDs and aspirin.

BE ALERT FOR OTC NSAID AND ASPIRIN USE
As with anticoagulants, combining OTC NSAIDs or aspirin with antiplatelet drugs can have harmful consequences. If a patient on antiplatelet therapy approaches the pharmacy counter to purchase an NSAID or aspirin, you should alert the pharmacist.

THE #1 SIDE EFFECT: BLEEDING
Bleeding associated with antiplatelet use can range from minor bleeding to life-threatening hemorrhage. Consequently, antiplatelets should not be used in patients with active pathological bleeding. Patients should report unusual bruising or bleeding to their healthcare provider.

STRESS THE IMPORTANCE OF TAKING EXACTLY AS PRESCRIBED
Compliance is important with all medications; however, the consequence of failing to take an antiplatelet as prescribed could be fatal. An overdose could cause a life-threatening hemorrhage, while missed doses could lead to a major event such as a heart attack or stroke.

VASODILATORS FOR ANGINA

BRAND NAME	GENERIC NAME
Apresoline®	Hydralazine
Imdur®	Isosorbide Mononitrate
Isordil®	Isosorbide Dinitrate
Nitro-Bid®	Nitroglycerin (topical ointment)
Nitro-Dur®	Nitroglycerin (transdermal patch)
Nitrostat®	Nitroglycerin (sublingual tablets)

BACKGROUND
Angina is severe chest pain caused by insufficient blood flow to the heart, and it can be the precursor to a heart attack.

PHARMACOLOGY
Expand blood vessels that supply blood to the heart.

INDICATIONS
Angina, Hypertension, Heart Failure

SIDE EFFECTS
Hypotension, Headache, Dizziness

DRUG INTERACTIONS
Increased risk of severe hypotension when used with other medications that can lower blood pressure (especially drugs like Viagra®, Cialis®, and Levitra®).

ACUTE ANGINA TREATMENT vs. PROPHYLAXIS
There are two ways to address angina: treatment and prevention. The only option listed above, and by far the most popular option, for treating acute angina is Nitrostat® (nitroglycerin sublingual tablets). The other drugs in the table above are for prophylaxis (i.e., prevention).

DISPENSING NITROSTAT®
The nitroglycerin in Nitrostat® is volatile, meaning it will evaporate if not stored properly. One of the storage requirements, according to the manufacturer drug package insert, is that the drug must be kept in the original glass vial at all times. For that reason, it is essential to dispense Nitrostat® in the original glass vial.

PATIENTS SHOULD TAKE NITROGLYCERIN WHILE SITTING DOWN
Nitroglycerin can cause hypotension and syncope. To avoid injury due to falling, the patient should sit down before taking a dose of nitroglycerin.

IMDUR® AND ISORDIL® ARE NOT EQUIVALENT
As their generic names suggest, Imdur® and Isordil® contain different amounts of nitrate. Imdur® (isosorbide mononitrate) contains one nitrate portion compared to the two contained in Isordil® (isosorbide dinitrate). In the body, nitrate is converted to nitric oxide, which relaxes and expands blood vessels. The mononitrate version of isosorbide is not interchangeable with the dinitrate version. Pharmacy technicians need to remember this when inputting prescriptions for isosorbide.

PHOSPHODIESTERASE-5 (PDE-5) INHIBITORS
FOR ERECTILE DYSFUNCTION

BRAND NAME	GENERIC NAME
Viagra®	Sildenafil
Cialis®	Tadalafil
Levitra®, Staxyn®	Vardenafil

Note: notice how the generic names of the PDE-5 Inhibitors end in "–afil."

BACKGROUND
A common cause of erectile dysfunction (male impotence) is insufficient blood flow to the penis.

PDE-5 INHIBITOR DRUG NAME STEM
-AFIL

PHARMACOLOGY
Prolong the activity of nitric oxide by blocking the enzyme (PDE-5) that deactivates nitric oxide. Nitric oxide is a potent vasodilator, so it expands blood vessels and increases blood flow. Since the enzyme, PDE-5 is predominantly present in the lungs and penis, these parts of the body are the beneficiaries of the effect. Increased blood flow to the penis leads to better, longer erections.

INDICATIONS
Erectile Dysfunction

SIDE EFFECTS
Headache, Hypotension, Priapism

DRUG INTERACTIONS
Increased risk of hypotension when used with other medications that expand blood vessels and/or lower blood pressure (especially nitroglycerin). Increased risk of epistaxis (nosebleed) when used with anticoagulant or antiplatelet drugs like Coumadin® and Plavix®.

CROSS SECTION OF A BLOOD VESSEL

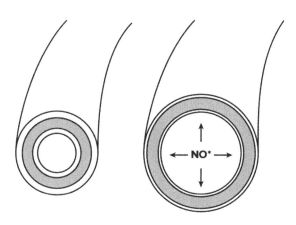

*NO = Nitric Oxide

ANTIARRHYTHMICS FOR CARDIAC ARRHYTHMIAS

BRAND NAME	GENERIC NAME
Pacerone®	Amiodarone
Lanoxin®	Digoxin
Norpace®	Disopyramide
Tikosyn®	Dofetilide
Tambocor®	Flecainide
Xylocaine®	Lidocaine
Rythmol®	Propafenone

BACKGROUND
Cardiac arrhythmias are caused by irregular nerve impulses that travel through the heart.

PHARMACOLOGY
Slow down/stabilize cardiac nerve impulses.

INDICATIONS
Cardiac Arrhythmias

SIDE EFFECTS
New (or Worsened) Cardiac Arrhythmias

DRUG INTERACTIONS
When taken with drugs that prolong the QT interval, life-threatening cardiac arrhythmias can result.

ANTIEMETICS FOR NAUSEA AND VOMITING

BRAND NAME	GENERIC NAME	
Zofran®	Ondansetron	Rx ONLY
Compazine®	Prochlorperazine	
Phenergan®	Promethazine	
Phenadoz®	Promethazine (suppository)	
Transderm-Scop®	Scopolamine (patch)	
Dramamine®	Dimenhydrinate	OTC
Antivert®, Bonine®, Dramamine® II	Meclizine	

BACKGROUND
Nausea and vomiting are associated with motion sickness, cancer chemotherapy, food poisoning, viral infections, and many other conditions and events. Nausea and vomiting are mediated by a variety of neurotransmitters, including acetylcholine, serotonin, histamine, and dopamine.

PHARMACOLOGY
There are several different classes of antiemetic drugs, each with a distinct mechanism of action, but those listed above work by blocking the action of one or more neurotransmitters. For example, Zofran® (ondansetron) works by blocking certain serotonin receptors associated with nausea and vomiting.

INDICATIONS
Nausea/Vomiting, Motion Sickness

SIDE EFFECTS
Drowsiness, Constipation

DRUG INTERACTIONS
Increased drowsiness when combined with opioids, benzodiazepines, alcohol, or other medications that cause drowsiness.

SELECTIVE SEROTONIN REUPTAKE INHIBITORS (SSRIs)
FOR DEPRESSION

BRAND NAME	GENERIC NAME
Celexa®	Citalopram
Lexapro®	Escitalopram
Prozac®	Fluoxetine
Luvox®	Fluvoxamine
Paxil®	Paroxetine
Zoloft®	Sertraline

BACKGROUND

Serotonin (chemical name: 5-hydroxytryptamine (5-HT)) is a neurotransmitter that plays a key role in depression, behavior, eating, and nausea/vomiting. Serotonin must be available in the synaptic cleft (the open space between neurons) long enough to exert an effect. When neurons reabsorb (or "reuptake") serotonin, the serotonin is removed from the synaptic cleft and is no longer in a location where it can exert its effect.

PHARMACOLOGY

Block the reuptake of serotonin, allowing serotonin to remain in the synaptic cleft where it has more time to exert its effect.

INDICATIONS

Depression, Behavior Disorders, Eating Disorders

SIDE EFFECTS

Changes in Body Weight, Nausea, Diarrhea, Serotonin Syndrome

DRUG INTERACTIONS

Increased risk of bleeding when used with NSAIDs, anticoagulants, or antiplatelets. Increased risk of serotonin syndrome when used with other medications that increase the effect of serotonin (e.g., SNRIs, TCAs).

NOTES

All antidepressants have the potential to cause suicidal ideation and behavior in young patients (ages 24 years and under. Patients should not abruptly stop taking an SSRI without consulting their physician).

SEVERAL WEEKS TO PEAK EFFECT

It is important to understand there are no quick fixes for depression.
All antidepressants have a slow onset of action and may require several weeks to reach peak effect.

SYMPTOMS OF SEROTONIN SYNDROME

Changes in mental status (e.g., agitation, confusion, hallucinations), pressured speech, tremor*, rigidity, diarrhea, fever, sweating, flushing, and seizures.

*Tremor is the hallmark symptom of serotonin syndrome.

SEROTONIN-NOREPINEPHRINE REUPTAKE INHIBITORS
(SNRIs) FOR DEPRESSION

BRAND NAME	GENERIC NAME
Pristiq®	Desvenlafaxine
Cymbalta®	Duloxetine
Savella®	Milnacipran
Effexor®	Venlafaxine

BACKGROUND
Similar to serotonin, norepinephrine also plays a role in depression and behavior.

PHARMACOLOGY
SNRIs work just like SSRIs, but in addition to blocking the reuptake of serotonin, they also block the reuptake of norepinephrine.

INDICATIONS
Depression, Eating Disorders, Anxiety Disorders, Diabetic Peripheral Neuropathy

SIDE EFFECTS
Side effects of SNRIs are similar to those of SSRIs (e.g., serotonin syndrome), but because they increase the effect of norepinephrine, they also have cardiovascular side effects (e.g., heart palpitations, hypertension, tachycardia).

DRUG INTERACTIONS
Increased risk of serotonin syndrome when taken with other drugs that increase serotonin activity (e.g., SSRIs, TCAs).

NOTES
All antidepressants have the potential to cause suicidal ideation and behavior in young patients (ages 24 years and under). Patients should not abruptly stop taking an SNRI without consulting their physician.

SEVERAL WEEKS TO PEAK EFFECT
It is important to understand there are no quick fixes for depression.
All antidepressants have a slow onset of action and may require several weeks to reach peak effect.

TRICYCLIC ANTIDEPRESSANTS (TCAs)
FOR DEPRESSION

BRAND NAME	GENERIC NAME
Elavil®	Amitriptyline
Sinequan®	Doxepin
Pamelor®	Nortriptyline
Tofranil®	Imipramine

BACKGROUND
Serotonin and norepinephrine play a role in mood and energy levels.

PHARMACOLOGY
Block the reuptake of serotonin and norepinephrine.

INDICATIONS
Depression, Eating Disorders, Generalized Anxiety Disorder, Diabetic Peripheral Neuropathy

SIDE EFFECTS
Tachycardia, Heart Palpitations, Hypertension, Dry Mouth, Weight Gain, Reduced Sex Drive, Serotonin Syndrome

DRUG INTERACTIONS
Increased risk of serotonin syndrome when taken with other drugs that increase serotonin activity (e.g., SSRIs, SNRIs).

NOTES
Tricyclic antidepressants are an older class of antidepressants. They generally have more side effects and drug interactions. SNRIs and TCAs are also occasionally prescribed for the treatment of certain kinds of pain. All antidepressants have the potential to cause suicidal ideation and behavior in young patients (ages 24 years and under). Patients should not abruptly stop taking a TCA without consulting their physician.

SEVERAL WEEKS TO PEAK EFFECT
It is important to understand there are no quick fixes for depression.
All antidepressants have a slow onset of action and may require several weeks to reach peak effect.

UNDERSTANDING DIABETES

DIABETES AND INSULIN

The human body is an organized collection of cells. Each cell uses glucose as the primary source of energy. Glucose is present in the blood, but cells need insulin to obtain glucose from the blood (see illustration below). In type II diabetes, the cells respond poorly to insulin, or the pancreas fails to secrete sufficient amounts of insulin. In either case, the cells are unable to consume glucose from the blood, and glucose builds up in the bloodstream. High levels of glucose in the blood have a damaging effect on blood vessels and nerve cells. Severe damage to blood vessels and neurons eventually leads to conditions like renal failure and blindness, which are typical consequences of poorly managed diabetes.

TYPE I vs. TYPE II DIABETES

As mentioned above, in type II diabetes, the cells respond poorly to insulin, or the pancreas fails to secrete the amount of insulin needed to maintain normal blood glucose levels. Patients with type II diabetes do not always require insulin injections. Many patients with type II diabetes can control their blood sugar with diet, exercise, and oral antidiabetics (e.g., metformin, sulfonylureas, DPP-4 inhibitors). Type I diabetes is different. In type I diabetes, the pancreas produces such little insulin that patients with this disease are not able to survive without insulin injections. In the United States, only 1 in 20 diabetic patients has type I diabetes. Type II diabetes is much more common, mainly due to the obesity epidemic.

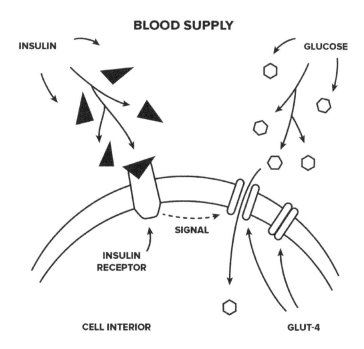

BLOOD SUPPLY

INSULIN   GLUCOSE

SIGNAL

INSULIN
RECEPTOR

CELL INTERIOR   GLUT-4

INSULIN FOR DIABETES

BRAND NAME	GENERIC NAME	
NovoLog®	Insulin Aspart	**Rx ONLY**
Tresiba®	Insulin Degludec	
Levemir®	Insulin Detemir	
Lantus®, Toujeo®	Insulin Glargine	
Apidra®	Insulin Glulisine	
Humalog®	Insulin Lispro	
Humalog 75/25®	Mixture of 75% Lispro Protamine Insulin and 25% Lispro Insulin	
Humulin R®, Novolin R®	Regular Human Insulin	**OTC**
Humulin N®, Novolin N®	Insulin NPH	
Novolin 70/30®, Humulin 70/30®	Mixture of 70% Insulin NPH and 30% Regular Human Insulin	

BACKGROUND
When food enters the intestinal tract, the nutrients are absorbed into the bloodstream. The body derives glucose, a type of sugar, from carbohydrate-containing foods and uses glucose as a source of energy.

PHARMACOLOGY
Stimulate cellular uptake of glucose from the blood. There are several different insulin formulations, each of which can be categorized based on how fast they start working (onset of action) and how long they work (duration of action).

CATEGORY	BRAND NAME	ONSET OF ACTION	DURATION OF ACTION
Rapid Acting	Apidra®, Humalog®, NovoLog®	15 - 30 min.	3 - 6 hours
Short Acting	Humulin R®, Novolin R®	30 - 60 min.	6 - 10 hours
Intermediate Acting	Humulin N®, Novolin N®	1 - 2 hours	16 - 24 hours
Long Acting	Lantus®, Levemir®, Toujeo®	1 - 2 hours	24 hours
Ultra Long Acting	Tresiba®	1 hour	24 - 40 hours

INDICATIONS
Type I Diabetes, Type II Diabetes

SIDE EFFECTS
Hypoglycemia, Redness/Swelling/Itching at the Injection Site

DRUG INTERACTIONS
Several drugs (e.g., thyroid hormones, diuretics, corticosteroids) can increase blood sugar, opposing the effect of insulin. Likewise, several medications (e.g., oral antidiabetics) can decrease blood sugar, increasing the risk of hypoglycemia.

NOTES
Keep refrigerated until dispensed. Most insulin expires after about 28 days at room temperature or after the rubber stopper of the vial is punctured. Except for U-500 insulin (Humulin® R U-500) and certain insulin pens (e.g., Toujeo®), the concentration of all insulin is standardized at 100 units per milliliter (each 0.01 mL contains 1 unit of insulin). Each milliliter of U-500 insulin (Humulin® R U-500) contains 500 units of insulin.

```
REFRIGERATE
DO NOT FREEZE
```

BIGUANIDES FOR DIABETES

BRAND NAME	GENERIC NAME
Glucophage®, Fortamet®	Metformin

BACKGROUND
Patients with diabetes have high blood glucose levels.

PHARMACOLOGY
Lowers blood glucose levels by three mechanisms:
1. Decreases the amount of glucose produced by the liver
2. Decreases intestinal absorption of glucose
3. Improves cellular response to insulin

Since metformin does not increase insulin secretion, it does not cause hypoglycemia, which (along with the fact that it is very cheap) is a big part of the reason metformin is so commonly prescribed.

INDICATIONS
Type II Diabetes

SIDE EFFECTS
Lactic Acidosis, Vitamin B12 Deficiency, Diarrhea, Nausea/Vomiting

DRUG INTERACTIONS
Tagamet® (cimetidine; an over the counter H_2 blocker for GERD) can increase metformin levels by up to 50%.

NOTES
Metformin is one of the most commonly prescribed diabetes medications. Do not be surprised if you see a patient who is on metformin getting a prescription for vitamin B12 injections (see side effects). Diarrhea, nausea, and vomiting are common during the first few days or weeks after beginning metformin, but patients develop a tolerance over time. Prescribers will often start patients on a low dose and increase to the optimal therapeutic dose over a few weeks. This strategy reduces the incidence of side effects for patients who have not yet developed a tolerance. For example, the instructions may look something like this:

Metformin 500 mg

Take one tablet by mouth once daily for one week, then one tablet twice daily for one week, then two tablets twice daily thereafter

If the patient started with two tablets twice daily right off the bat, the initial blood glucose-lowering effect would be better, but there would be a higher likelihood of diarrhea, nausea, and vomiting, and consequently, the patient would be less likely to continue taking the medication due to the unpleasant side effects.

EXTENDED RELEASE METFORMIN HAS FEWER SIDE EFFECTS

Extended release formulations of metformin are more expensive, but they are associated with fewer side effects, particularly the gastrointestinal side effects (i.e., diarrhea, nausea, and vomiting) that tend to be so bothersome with the immediate release formulation. Despite the higher cost, some prescribers prefer to prescribe extended release metformin for this reason.

SULFONYLUREAS FOR DIABETES

BRAND NAME	GENERIC NAME
Amaryl®	Glimepiride
Glucotrol®	Glipizide
DiaBeta®, Micronase®	Glyburide

BACKGROUND
The pancreas secretes Insulin, but in type II diabetes, the pancreas may fail to secrete sufficient amounts of insulin.

PHARMACOLOGY
Stimulate the pancreas to secrete insulin.

INDICATIONS
Type II Diabetes

SIDE EFFECTS
Hypoglycemia, Weight Gain

TAKE WITH FOOD

DRUG INTERACTIONS
Many drugs can increase the risk of hypoglycemia. Likewise, several drugs can reduce the effect of sulfonylureas.

NOTES
Another term for the sulfonylurea is "secretagogue," because they stimulate insulin secretion.

DIPEPTIDYL PEPTIDASE-4 (DPP-4) INHIBITORS
FOR DIABETES

BRAND NAME	GENERIC NAME
Nesina®	Alogliptin
Tradjenta®	Linagliptin
Onglyza®	Saxagliptin
Januvia®	Sitagliptin

Note: notice how the generic names of the DPP-4 Inhibitors end "–gliptin."

BACKGROUND
Naturally present in the human body, incretins are hormones that signal the pancreas to increase insulin release.

DPP-4 INHIBITOR DRUG NAME STEM
-GLIPTIN

PHARMACOLOGY
Delay the breakdown of incretins, thus increasing their activity. Increased incretin activity leads to increased insulin secretion.

INDICATIONS
Type II Diabetes

SIDE EFFECTS
Hypoglycemia, Muscle Pain, SJS (rare)

DRUG INTERACTIONS
Increased risk of hypoglycemia when used with other diabetes medications.

GLUCAGON-LIKE PEPTIDE-1 (GLP-1) AGONISTS
FOR DIABETES

BRAND NAME	GENERIC NAME
Byetta®, Bydureon®	Exenatide
Trulicity®	Dulaglutide
Victoza®	Liraglutide

BACKGROUND
Incretins are hormones that are naturally produced by the body. They signal the pancreas to increase insulin release.

PHARMACOLOGY
Mimic incretins to signal the pancreas to increase insulin release.

INDICATIONS
Type II Diabetes

SIDE EFFECTS
Nausea/Vomiting, Diarrhea, Constipation

DRUG INTERACTIONS
Increased risk of hypoglycemia when used with other diabetes medications.

NOTES
Manufacturers supply GLP-1 agonists in pens for injection. It is important to keep the medication refrigerated until dispensed. According to the package inserts, Victoza® and Byetta® should be discarded after 30 days at room temperature or 30 days after the first use, whichever comes first. Bydureon® should be discarded after 28 days at room temperature or 30 days after the first use, whichever comes first. Trulicity, a once-weekly single-use pen, may be stored at room temperature for up to 14 days.

GLP-1 AGONISTS SHOULD BE ADMINISTERED BY SUBCUTANEOUS INJECTION ONLY

ROUTE OF ADMINISTRATION
GLP-1 agonists are peptides (short-chain amino acids), which the digestive tract indiscriminately digests. However, for these medications to exert the intended pharmacologic effect, they must maintain their chemical structure, which means they cannot be administered orally. They must be injected.

REFRIGERATE
DO NOT FREEZE

UNDERSTANDING ACID REFLUX

The stomach contains strong acid, and this acid has two essential functions. First, it kills bacteria, preventing infectious organisms from entering the body. Second, it begins the process of breaking down and digesting food. The stomach has mechanisms to protect itself from the corrosive effects of acid, but the esophagus does not. Acid reflux, or heartburn, occurs when acid from the stomach overflows or splashes up into the esophagus (see illustration). Most people experience heartburn on an occasional basis, usually after consuming spicy or greasy food, but other people can experience heartburn more frequently. Physicians may diagnose these individuals with a condition known as Gastroesophageal Reflux Disease (GERD). GERD is a chronic condition. Over time, the acid can severely damage the esophagus and cause serious problems.

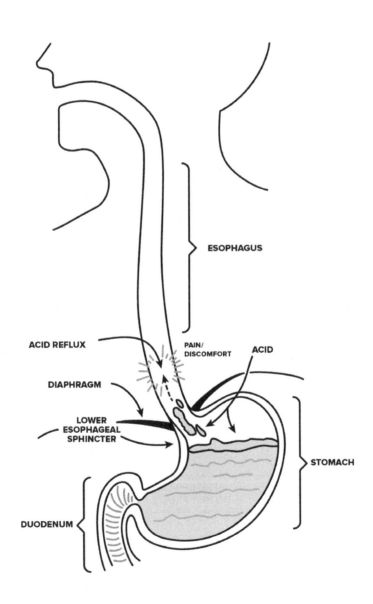

ANTACIDS FOR ACID REFLUX

BRAND NAME	GENERIC NAME	
Gaviscon®	Aluminum Hydroxide/Magnesium Carbonate	OTC
Mylanta®	Aluminum Hydroxide/Magnesium Carbonate/Simethicone	
Rolaids®	Calcium Carbonate/Magnesium Hydroxide	
Tums®, Maalox®	Calcium Carbonate	

BACKGROUND
Bases neutralize acids.

PHARMACOLOGY
Neutralize stomach acid, converting the acid to water.

INDICATIONS
Heartburn, Upset Stomach

SIDE EFFECTS
Constipation (Calcium and Aluminum), Diarrhea (Magnesium), Kidney Stones (Calcium)

DRUG INTERACTIONS
Antacids interfere with the absorption of certain medications. Most interactions can be avoided by separating the administration by at least two hours.

BELCHING, BLOATING, and FLATULENCE

Calcium carbonate is unique. The reaction between calcium carbonate ($CaCO_3$) and hydrochloric acid (HCl) yields water (H_2O), carbon dioxide (CO_2), and calcium chloride ($CaCl_2$).

$$CaCO_3 + HCl \Rightarrow H_2O + CO_2 + CaCl_2$$

Acid neutralized. Mission accomplished, right? Yes, but not without consequences. As we know, carbon dioxide is a gas. So, the most common side effects of calcium carbonate are perhaps exactly what you would expect—belching, bloating, and flatulence.

SIMETHICONE

Simethicone is a surface-active agent (or "surfactant") similar to a detergent. It breaks the surface tension on gas bubbles in the gastrointestinal tract, providing relief from bloating, gas pains, and flatulence.

ANTACID SIDE EFFECTS ACCORDING TO ELEMENTAL CONTENT

	Constipation	Diarrhea	Kidney Stones
Aluminum	✓		
Calcium	✓		✓
Magnesium		✓	

HISTAMINE-2 RECEPTOR ANTAGONISTS (H2 BLOCKERS)
FOR ACID REFLUX

BRAND NAME	GENERIC NAME	
Tagamet®	Cimetidine	
Pepcid®	Famotidine	OTC
Axid®	Nizatidine	
Zantac®	Ranitidine	

Note: notice how the generic names of the H$_2$-blockers end "–tidine."

BACKGROUND

Histamine binds to H2 receptors and increases stomach acid production.

> **H2 BLOCKER** DRUG NAME STEM
> ## -TIDINE

PHARMACOLOGY

H2 blockers prevent histamine from binding to H2 receptors, thus reducing stomach acid production.

INDICATIONS

Heartburn, Gastroesophageal Reflux Disease (GERD)

SIDE EFFECTS

Constipation, Gynecomastia (cimetidine only)

DRUG INTERACTIONS

Some drugs rely on stomach acid for absorption, and, since H2 blockers reduce stomach acid, absorption of other drugs may be impaired.

ONSET *of* ACTION

With an onset of action occurring within 60 minutes of administration, H2 blockers begin working faster than proton pump inhibitors (PPIs).

CIMETIDINE-INDUCED GYNECOMASTIA

Gynecomastia is a condition characterized by enlarged breast tissue in boys and men. Although rare, Tagamet® (cimetidine) is well-known for its potential to cause drug-induced gynecomastia.

OVER-THE-COUNTER AVAILABILITY

Zantac® (ranitidine 75 mg & 150 mg), Pepcid® AC (famotidine 10 & 20 mg), Tagamet® (cimetidine 200 mg), and Axid® AR (nizatidine 75 mg) are available over the counter. Higher strengths are available by prescription only. As with PPIs, patients should not use over the counter H2 blockers for more than 14 days without consulting a healthcare provider.

PROTON PUMP INHIBITORS (PPIs)
FOR ACID REFLUX

BRAND NAME	GENERIC NAME	
Dexilant®	Dexlansoprazole	Rx
Protonix®	Pantoprazole	
Nexium®	Esomeprazole	OTC
Prevacid®	Lansoprazole	
Prilosec®	Omeprazole	
AciPhex®	Rabeprazole	

Note: notice how the generic names of the PPIs end "–prazole."

PPI DRUG NAME STEM
-PRAZOLE

BACKGROUND
Structures in the stomach known as "proton pumps" are responsible for producing acid.

PHARMACOLOGY
Proton pump inhibitors interfere with the function of proton pumps, thus decreasing the amount of acid in the stomach.

INDICATIONS
Heartburn, Gastroesophageal Reflux Disease (GERD)

SIDE EFFECTS
Abdominal Pain, Diarrhea, Nausea/Vomiting, Bone Fractures

DRUG INTERACTIONS
As with other acid-reducing medications, PPIs may interfere with the absorption of certain drugs that rely on stomach acid for absorption.

PATIENT SHOULD TAKE BEFORE A MEAL FOR THE BEST RESULTS
PPIs must be introduced into an acidic environment to be activated. Ingestion of food stimulates gastric acid production. For this reason, PPIs generally work best when taken before a meal.

OVER THE COUNTER AVAILABILITY
Prilosec OTC® (omeprazole 20 mg), Nexium® 24 HR (esomeprazole 20 mg), and Prevacid® 24 HR (lansoprazole 15 mg) are each available over the counter. Dexilant® (dexlansoprazole), Protonix (pantoprazole), and higher strengths of the other PPIs are available by prescription only. Due to the potential for long-term side effects, patients should not use over-the-counter PPIs for more than 14 days without consulting a healthcare provider.

ANTI-EPILEPTIC DRUGS (AEDs)
FOR SEIZURES

BRAND NAME		GENERIC NAME
Tegretol®, Epitol®		Carbamazepine
Depakote®		Divalproex
Neurontin®		Gabapentin
Vimpat®	C-V	Lacosamide
Lamictal®		Lamotrigine
Keppra®		Levetiracetam
Trileptal®		Oxcarbazepine
Dilantin®		Phenytoin
Lyrica®	C-V	Pregabalin
Topamax®		Topiramate
Zonegran®		Zonisamide

BACKGROUND
Seizures are caused by abnormal, hyperactive nerve function.

PHARMACOLOGY
AEDs work by suppressing nerve activity. There are various mechanisms by which this is accomplished (e.g., sodium ion channel modulation, gamma-aminobutyric acid (GABA)* receptor stimulation, glutamate** receptor antagonism).

> * GABA is the primary *inhibitory* neurotransmitter of the central nervous system. It slows things down.
> ** Glutamate is the primary *excitatory* neurotransmitter of the central nervous system.

INDICATIONS
Seizures, Nerve Pain, Psychiatric Disorders

SIDE EFFECTS
Drowsiness, Mental Slowness, Weight Gain, Rash, SJS (rare)

DRUG INTERACTIONS
Severe nervous system suppression when combined with other drugs that suppress the nervous system (e.g., benzodiazepines, opioids, alcohol).

NOTES
Anti-epileptic drugs are also referred to as anticonvulsants.

PATIENTS SHOULD NOT DISCONTINUE ABRUPTLY
Compliance is essential for antiepileptic drugs. Abrupt discontinuation can lead to status epilepticus with potentially fatal hypoxia. These medications must be taken exactly as prescribed.

ANTIBIOTICS FOR BACTERIAL INFECTIONS

BRAND NAME	GENERIC NAME
Amoxil®	Amoxicillin
Augmentin®	Amoxicillin/Clavulanate
Bactrim®, Septra®	Sulfamethoxazole/Trimethoprim
Keflex®	Cephalexin
Cipro®	Ciprofloxacin
Biaxin®	Clarithromycin

BRAND NAME	GENERIC NAME
Levaquin®	Levofloxacin
Flagyl®	Metronidazole
Avelox®	Moxifloxacin
Veetids®	Penicillin
Zithromax®, Z-Pak®	Azithromycin
Vancocin®	Vancomycin

BACKGROUND
There are several structural and physiological differences between human cells and bacterial cells.

PHARMACOLOGY
There are many different classes of antibiotics, each with a distinct mechanism of action, but every antibiotic works on a basic level by exploiting a difference between bacterial cells and human cells. For instance, clarithromycin kills living cells by binding to a structure that is only present in bacterial cells, leaving human cells unaffected.

INDICATIONS
Bacterial Infections

FINISH ALL MEDICATION
UNLESS DIRECTED OTHERWISE

SIDE EFFECTS
Diarrhea

DRUG INTERACTIONS
Antibiotics increase the effect of warfarin, which increases the risk of bleeding. They may also decrease the effect of oral contraceptives.

IMPORTANT EDUCATION POINTS FOR ANTIBIOTICS
#1 Antibiotics should only be used for bacterial infections. They are not effective for viral or fungal infections.
#2 To prevent the development of antibiotic-resistant bacteria, patients should finish the entire prescribed course of antibiotics. Advise patients not to discontinue the antibiotics early, even if they feel better.
#3 In killing pathogenic bacteria, antibiotics also kill good bacteria (flora), including the good bacteria that normally colonize the gastrointestinal tract. This commonly results in diarrhea, nausea, and vomiting–the most common side effects of antibiotics–and potential overgrowth of *Clostridium difficile* leading to *C. difficile*-associated diarrhea (CDAD), which can be potentially fatal. If the patient develops symptoms of CDAD, such as watery and bloody stools, they should notify their physician.
#4 Intestinal flora produce vitamin K that is absorbed into the bloodstream, so antibiotics can be expected to reduce vitamin K levels. In the presence of less vitamin K, warfarin exerts a stronger anticoagulant effect that can lead to severe bleeding events. Patients on warfarin may need to be monitored more closely by their physician while receiving antibiotics.

PRECAUTIONARY MEASURE TO PREVENT CROSS-CONTAMINATION
Patients commonly report allergies to penicillin and sulfa antibiotics. In some cases, those allergies are severe and life-threatening. To prevent cross-contamination, clean the counting tray and spatula with 70% isopropyl alcohol (or similar) after counting drugs like sulfamethoxazole/trimethoprim or penicillin to remove any visible or invisible medication residue that may be left behind. Alternatively, some pharmacies designate separate spatulas and counting trays for these medications.

CORTICOSTEROIDS FOR INFLAMMATION

BRAND NAME	GENERIC NAME
Cortef®	Hydrocortisone
Sterapred®	Prednisone
Orapred®	Prednisolone
Medrol®	Methylprednisolone
Decadron®	Dexamethasone

Note: notice how the generic names of the corticosteroids end "–sone" or "solone."

BACKGROUND
Activation of glucocorticoid receptors reduces the production of inflammatory mediators and suppresses immune system activity.

CORTICOSTEROID DRUG NAME STEMS
-SONE   -SOLONE

PHARMACOLOGY
Corticosteroids bind to and activate glucocorticoid receptors.

INDICATIONS
Inflammation, Allergic Reactions, Autoimmune Disorders, Adrenal Insufficiency

SIDE EFFECTS
Gastrointestinal (GI) Irritation/Ulceration, Fluid Retention, Hypertension, Hyperglycemia, Weight Gain, Thinning of the Skin (topical corticosteroids)

> **NOTE:** The likelihood and severity of side effects increase with dose and duration of treatment.

DRUG INTERACTIONS
Antibiotics increase the effect of warfarin, which increases the risk of bleeding. They may also decrease the effect of oral contraceptives.

ADMINISTER WITH FOOD OR MILK TO REDUCE GI IRRITATION AND PEPTIC ULCER RISK

POTENTIAL CONSEQUENCES OF IMMUNOSUPPRESSION

IMPAIRED WOUND HEALING	INCREASED SUSCEPTIBILITY TO INFECTION	MASKING OF SIGNS OF INFECTION

NOTE: Patients receiving immunosuppressive doses of corticosteroids cannot receive certain vaccines.

CORTICOSTEROID WITHDRAWAL
The body produces about 20 mg of hydrocortisone ("cortisol") daily at baseline. High doses of medicinal corticosteroids suppress physiologic cortisol production. Once this occurs, abrupt discontinuation of the corticosteroid can trigger withdrawal symptoms (e.g., fever, muscle aches, joint pain, malaise). To reduce the likelihood of withdrawal symptoms, the dose should be tapered (i.e., gradually decreased) over several days.

CONSIDERATIONS FOR TOPICAL STEROIDS

THINNING OF THE SKIN	SYSTEMIC ABSORPTION
The most common side effect associated with topical steroids, particularly with chronic use, is thinning of the skin at the application site.	To reduce systemic absorption, the application site should not be covered (e.g., with bandages or wraps) unless the physician instructs otherwise.

NON-STEROIDAL ANTI-INFLAMMATORY DRUGS (NSAIDs)
FOR PAIN/INFLAMMATION

BRAND NAME	GENERIC NAME	
Celebrex®	Celecoxib	**Rx ONLY**
Voltaren®	Diclofenac	
Indocin®	Indomethacin	
Lodine®	Etodolac	
Mobic®	Meloxicam	
Relafen®	Nabumetone	
Toradol®	Ketorolac	
Aleve®, Naprosyn®	Naproxen	**OTC**
Bayer Aspirin Extra Strength®	Aspirin	
Motrin®, Advil®	Ibuprofen	

BACKGROUND
Inflammation commonly causes pain. The process of inflammation is mediated by prostaglandins, which are naturally produced within the body.

PHARMACOLOGY
Block cyclooxygenase (COX), the enzyme responsible for the production of prostaglandins.

INDICATIONS
Pain, Inflammation, Fever

SIDE EFFECTS
Nausea and Vomiting, Stomach Ulcers, Renal Impairment, Cardiovascular Events (excluding low-dose aspirin, which can actually be used to prevent cardiovascular events), Reye's Syndrome (aspirin only)

DRUG INTERACTIONS
Increased risk of bleeding (especially gastrointestinal bleeding) when used with anticoagulant or antiplatelet drugs.

NOTES
Prostaglandins also play a key role in protecting the lining of the stomach from acid-related damage. Since NSAIDs reduce prostaglandin production, short-term NSAID use can cause nausea and upset stomach; meanwhile, long-term use can lead to stomach ulcers. To reduce these side effects, we often recommend taking NSAIDs with food. Also, worth noting, aspirin is a little different from the other NSAIDs. Aspirin not only has anti-inflammatory effects but also antiplatelet effects (i.e., aspirin helps prevent blood clot formation). For that reason, aspirin may be prescribed for heart attack and stroke prevention.

AVOID NSAIDs DURING THE THIRD TRIMESTER OF PREGNANCY
The use of NSAIDs by women ≥ 30 weeks pregnant can cause premature closure of the fetal ductus arteriosus, a potentially deadly cardiovascular defect.

THE 5-DAY LIMIT FOR TORADOL® (KETOROLAC)
Toradol® (ketorolac) is the most potent NSAID. While other NSAIDs can be used for mild-moderate pain, Toradol® is approved for moderately severe acute pain; however, this power comes with drawbacks. Toradol® should only be used short-term (**no more than 5 days**) due to a higher risk of potentially severe gastrointestinal bleeding and renal toxicity.

OPIOIDS FOR PAIN

BRAND NAME		GENERIC NAME
various combination products*	C-III – C-V	Codeine†
various combination products**	C-II	Hydrocodone
Dilaudid®	C-II	Hydromorphone
MS Contin®, Kadian®	C-II	Morphine (extended release)
Roxanol®	C-II	Morphine (immediate release)
Oxycontin®	C-II	Oxycodone (extended release)
Roxicodone®	C-II	Oxycodone (immediate release)
Ultram®	C-IV	Tramadol

* Robitussin® AC, Tylenol® #3   ** Norco®, Lortab®, Tussionex®, Tussigon®
†Codeine by itself (not in a combination formulation) is a C-II

BACKGROUND
Activation of opioid receptors produces analgesia and sedation.

PHARMACOLOGY
Activate opioid receptors, providing pain relief.

INDICATIONS
Pain, Cough (codeine and hydrocodone)

SIDE EFFECTS
Sedation, Respiratory Depression, Constipation, Dependency

> MAY CAUSE DROWSINESS

DRUG INTERACTIONS
Increased incidence of sedation and respiratory depression when taken with other drugs that suppress the central nervous system (e.g., benzodiazepines, alcohol).

THE OPIUM POPPY PLANT
Morphine and codeine are compounds derived directly from the opium poppy. Hydro**morph**one and oxy**morph**one are semi-synthetic derivatives of morphine. Hydro**cod**one and oxy**cod**one are semi-synthetic derivatives of codeine. Opioids like fentanyl and methadone are fully synthetic (i.e., man-made).

CONTROLLED SUBSTANCES
All opioid analgesics are categorized as controlled substances due to their potential for abuse and addiction.

OPIOID WITHDRAWAL SYMPTOMS
For patients on opioids long-term, abrupt discontinuation can cause severe withdrawal symptoms. In these patients, the opioid must be discontinued gradually over time to avoid withdrawal.

OPIOID-INDUCED CONSTIPATION
Constipation is the only side effect to which patients do not develop a tolerance. As the dose of the opioid increases, constipation worsens. Patients receiving opioids long-term usually need daily laxatives.

THE ANTIDOTE FOR OPIOIDS
Narcan® (naloxone), an opioid receptor antagonist.

BENZODIAZEPINES FOR ANXIETY

BRAND NAME		GENERIC NAME
Xanax®	C-IV	Alprazolam
Librium®	C-IV	Chlordiazepoxide
Onfi®	C-IV	Clobazam
Klonopin®	C-IV	Clonazepam
Valium®, Diastat®	C-IV	Diazepam
Ativan®	C-IV	Lorazepam
Versed®	C-IV	Midazolam
Restoril®	C-IV	Temazepam
Halcion®	C-IV	Triazolam

Note: notice how the generic names of most of the benzodiazepines end in "–azepam" or "-azolam."

BACKGROUND

There are two benzodiazepine receptor subtypes – BNZ_1 and BNZ_2. BNZ_1 receptor activation promotes sleep; meanwhile, BNZ_2 receptor activation promotes muscle relaxation.

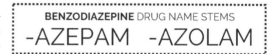

BENZODIAZEPINE DRUG NAME STEMS
-AZEPAM   -AZOLAM

PHARMACOLOGY

Benzodiazepines bind to benzodiazepine receptors (BNZ_1 and BNZ_2) and enhance the effect of gamma-aminobutyric acid (GABA), the primary inhibitory neurotransmitter of the central nervous system. These effects can be useful in the treatment of anxiety, insomnia, muscle spasms, seizures, and other conditions.

INDICATIONS

Anxiety, Insomnia, Agitation, Seizures, Muscle Spasms, Alcohol Withdrawal

SIDE EFFECTS

Drowsiness, Somnolence, Dependency

MAY CAUSE DROWSINESS

DRUG INTERACTIONS

Increased drowsiness when used with other drugs that suppress the central nervous system (e.g., sedative-hypnotics, opioids, anticonvulsants, alcohol).

C-IV

CONTROLLED SUBSTANCES

Due to their mild potential for abuse and addiction, all benzodiazepines are classified as Schedule IV controlled substances according to federal law.

PATIENTS SHOULD NOT DISCONTINUE ABRUPTLY

Dependence can develop quickly. Abrupt discontinuation may precipitate severe withdrawal symptoms, including seizures. Benzodiazepines should be discontinued gradually. Patients should not stop taking a benzodiazepine without first consulting with their physician.

THE ANTIDOTE for BENZODIAZEPINES

Romazicon® (flumazenil), a benzodiazepine receptor antagonist.

SEDATIVE-HYPNOTICS FOR INSOMNIA

BRAND NAME		GENERIC NAME
Lunesta®	C-IV	Eszopiclone
Sonata®	C-IV	Zaleplon
Ambien®	C-IV	Zolpidem

BACKGROUND
The BNZ$_1$ benzodiazepine receptor can be activated by gamma-aminobutyric acid (GABA), the chief inhibitory neurotransmitter of the central nervous system. Activation of the BNZ$_1$ receptor promotes sleep.

PHARMACOLOGY
Bind to the GABA-benzodiazepine receptor complex, enhancing the effect of GABA to promote sleep.

INDICATIONS
Insomnia

SIDE EFFECTS
Drowsiness, Somnolence, Dependency

MAY CAUSE DROWSINESS

DRUG INTERACTIONS
Increased drowsiness when used with other drugs that suppress central nervous system activity (e.g., benzodiazepines, opioids, antihistamines, alcohol).

NOTES
All drugs in this class are Schedule IV controlled substances.

C-IV
CONTROLLED SUBSTANCES
Eszopiclone, zaleplon, and zolpidem each have a mild potential for abuse and addiction.

DEVOTE A FULL NIGHT TO SLEEP
The sedative-hypnotic effect typically wears off after approximately eight hours or less. Consequently, these medications should only be used when the patient can devote a full night (about 7–8 hours) to sleep. Patients should also be warned of the potential for "next-day impairment" (i.e., daytime drowsiness that may preclude them from safely operating a vehicle the day after using the medication).

SLEEP-WALKING AND OTHER COMPLEX BEHAVIORS
Non-benzodiazepine sedative-hypnotics have been associated with sleep-walking, sleep-driving, making phone calls, and preparing and eating food while not fully awake and with no memory afterward.

STIMULANTS FOR ADHD

BRAND NAME		GENERIC NAME
Adderall®	C-II	Amphetamine/Dextroamphetamine
Strattera®		Atomoxetine
Kapvay®		Clonidine
Focalin®	C-II	Dexmethylphenidate
Intuniv®		Guanfacine
Vyvanse®	C-II	Lisdexamfetamine
Daytrana®	C-II	Methylphenidate (patch)
Ritalin®	C-II	Methylphenidate
Concerta®	C-II	Methylphenidate (extended release)

BACKGROUND
A major symptom of Attention Deficit Hyperactivity Disorder (ADHD) is poor mental focus.

PHARMACOLOGY
Stimulate the central nervous system (i.e., the brain), thereby improving mental focus.

INDICATIONS
ADHD, Narcolepsy

SIDE EFFECTS
Insomnia, Hypertension, Dependency

DRUG INTERACTIONS
Use with other stimulants, such as caffeine and weight-loss drugs, increases the risk of high blood pressure and cardiovascular problems.

ADMINISTER IN THE MORNING
Evening or nighttime administration is likely to cause insomnia.

UNDERSTANDING ASTHMA AND COPD

LUNG DISEASE AND CONSTRICTED AIRWAYS

Asthma and Chronic Obstructive Pulmonary Disease (COPD) are characterized by poor lung function and difficulty breathing. One of the primary ways we can treat these diseases is with drugs that expand/dilate the airways, making it easier for patients to breathe. There are two types of receptors relevant to this conversation: beta-receptors, activation of which stimulates airway dilation, and acetylcholine receptors, activation of which stimulates airway constriction.

BETA-RECEPTORS

Substances such as epinephrine and norepinephrine activate beta-receptors. In the airways, activation of these receptors leads to airway expansion/ dilation. For lung diseases such as asthma and COPD, this effect can be very therapeutic. Consequently, many asthma and COPD drugs are beta-receptor agonists.

ACETYLCHOLINE RECEPTORS

In the lungs, acetylcholine receptor activation causes the airways to constrict, which makes breathing difficult for patients with lung disease. For that reason, we use drugs that block or prevent the activation of acetylcholine receptors. These are called acetylcholine receptor antagonists, or "anticholinergics."

INFLAMMATION

Besides airway constriction, inflammation is also associated with asthma and COPD. For that reason, practitioners frequently prescribe inhaled corticosteroids to suppress airway inflammation in these patients.

THE USE OF INHALED DOSAGE FORMS

Most of the drugs used to treat asthma and COPD are manufactured as inhaled dosage forms, such as nebulizer solutions, metered dose inhalers, and dry powder inhalers. These dosage forms allow the medication to be delivered directly to the site of action inside the lungs. When a drug is taken systemically (e.g., orally or by injection), it enters the bloodstream and travels to all areas of the body, which can cause many side effects. When a drug is applied locally, directly to the site of action, as is the case with inhaled dosage forms in the treatment of lung disease, this not only maximizes the effectiveness of the medication but also minimizes side effects because it prevents other areas of the body from being exposed to the drug.

INHALED BETA AGONISTS
FOR ASTHMA AND COPD

BRAND NAME	GENERIC NAME	
ProAir®, Proventil®, Ventolin® HFA	Albuterol (inhaler)	**SHORT ACTING**
AccuNeb®	Albuterol (nebulizer solution)	
Xopenex® HFA	Levalbuterol (inhaler)	
Xopenex®	Levalbuterol (nebulizer solution)	
Brovana®	Arformoterol (nebulizer solution)	**LONG ACTING**
Foradil Aerolizer®	Formoterol (inhaler)	
Perforomist®	Formoterol (inhaler)	
Serevent®	Salmeterol (diskus/inhaler)	

BACKGROUND
One of the main problems in asthma and COPD is narrowed airways. When beta-receptors in the lungs are activated, the airways dilate.

PHARMACOLOGY
Activate beta-receptors in the lungs to dilate the airways, making it easier for patients to breathe.

INDICATIONS
Asthma, COPD

FOR INHALATION ONLY

SIDE EFFECTS
Tachycardia, Palpitations

DRUG INTERACTIONS
Certain beta-blockers (e.g., carvedilol) can oppose the effect of inhaled beta agonists.

NOTES
There are two classes of inhaled beta agonists – short acting and long acting. Patients usually use short acting beta agonists for asthma attacks; thus, the term "rescue inhaler" is used for albuterol inhalers. The typical asthma patient only uses short acting beta agonists on an "as needed" basis, not on a schedule. On the other hand, prescribers employ long acting beta agonists to prevent symptoms of asthma or COPD. Long acting beta agonists are not effective for acute asthma attacks, and they are used on a scheduled daily basis.

ROUTE OF ADMINISTRATION: ADVANTAGES AND DISADVANTAGES

Administration by inhalation delivers the drug directly to the site of action (the lungs), which maximizes the therapeutic effect while minimizing side effects. However, for an inhaler to be effective, the patient must be able to press the actuator and inhale deeply at the same time. For patients with poor coordination, attaching a spacer to the mouthpiece can solve this problem.

CARDIOVASCULAR SIDE EFFECTS

Beta$_2$ receptors are found predominantly in the lungs; however, receptor selectivity is never 100%. Some minor beta$_1$ receptor activation (located predominantly in the heart) also occurs, which can result in side effects like tachycardia and palpitations.

INHALED ANTICHOLINERGICS
FOR ASTHMA AND COPD

BRAND NAME	GENERIC NAME
Atrovent®	Ipratropium (nebulizer solution)
Atrovent® HFA	Ipratropium (inhaler)
Spiriva® Respimat	Tiotropium (inhaler)
Spiriva® HandiHaler	Tiotropium (capsules for inhalation)

SHORT-ACTING	LONG-ACTING
Atrovent® (ipratropium)	Spiriva® (tiotropium)

BACKGROUND

As with asthma, one of the main problems in COPD is narrowed airways. Activation of acetylcholine receptors in the lungs leads to airway constriction/narrowing.

PHARMACOLOGY

Block activation of acetylcholine receptors, thereby reducing airway constriction.

INDICATIONS

COPD

FOR INHALATION ONLY

SIDE EFFECTS

Dry Mouth, Constipation

DRUG INTERACTIONS

For patients experiencing constipation from opioid uses, the addition of an inhaled anticholinergic drug can worsen this constipation.

NOTES

Ipratropium (a short acting anticholinergic) is usually taken four times daily; whereas, tiotropium (long acting) must be taken only once daily. Anticholinergics are not effective in treating acute asthma symptoms ("asthma attacks").

WARNING FOR SPIRIVA® HANDIHALER®

The capsules that come with the Spiriva® Handihaler® device should never be swallowed. The Handihaler® device is designed to puncture the capsule, allowing the powder inside the capsule can be inhaled.

COMBINED ANTICHOLINERGICS AND SHORT-ACTING BETA AGONISTS

Since the inhaled beta agonists and inhaled anticholinergics have a different mechanism of action, practitioners commonly prescribe both drugs for simultaneous use. For that reason, manufacturers developed a combination albuterol and ipratropium inhaler and nebulizer solution (see below).

BRAND NAME	GENERIC NAME
Combivent Respimat®	Ipratropium/Albuterol (inhaler)
DuoNeb®	Ipratropium/Albuterol (nebulizer solution)

INHALED CORTICOSTEROIDS
FOR ASTHMA AND COPD

BRAND NAME	GENERIC NAME
Asmanex®	Mometasone
Flovent®	Fluticasone
Pulmicort®	Budesonide
Qvar®	Beclomethasone

BACKGROUND
Inflammation plays a major role in asthma and COPD.

PHARMACOLOGY
Block the body's natural mechanism for the production of inflammatory mediators, thus reducing inflammation.

INDICATIONS
Asthma, COPD

SIDE EFFECTS
Oral Thrush, Upper Respiratory Infection, Sinusitis

RINSE MOUTH AFTER USE

DRUG INTERACTIONS
Certain drugs can increase or decrease the activity of corticosteroids.

NOTES
For inhaled corticosteroid prescriptions, many practitioners include the instructions: "rinse mouth after use." Rinsing is necessary because corticosteroid residue left in the mouth can cause oral thrush, a fungal infection in the mouth.

MUST BE USED CONSISTENTLY ON A DAILY BASIS

Inhaled corticosteroids should be used daily for maintenance treatment. They are effective for symptom prevention, but they are not effective for acute bronchospasm ("asthma attacks"). Missed doses increase the risk of asthma attacks and may lead to a general worsening of symptoms.

RINSE MOUTH AFTER EACH USE

Inhaled corticosteroids are potent anti-inflammatory drugs. Inevitably, they encounter the oral cavity en route to the lungs, suppressing immune system activity within the oral cavity and opening the door to issues like oral thrush (a fungal infection of the mouth). To reduce the incidence of oral thrush, instruct each patient to rinse their mouth with water after each use.

COMBINED CORTICOSTEROIDS AND LONG-ACTING BETA AGONISTS

The pathophysiology of asthma includes bronchial smooth muscle constriction, airway inflammation, and bronchial hyperresponsiveness. While corticosteroids have potent anti-inflammatory effects, they do not treat the underlying bronchoconstriction. For this reason, inhaled corticosteroids are commonly combined with a long-acting beta$_2$ agonist. Examples include Advair® (fluticasone/salmeterol), Dulera® (mometasone/formoterol), and Symbicort® (budesonide/formoterol).

ANTIHISTAMINES
FOR ALLERGIES

BRAND NAME	GENERIC NAME	
Benadryl® Dramamine® Unisom®	Diphenhydramine Dimenhydrinate Doxylamine	**OTC**
Allegra® Claritin® Zyrtec®	Fexofenadine Loratadine Cetirizine	

BACKGROUND
Histamine is associated with symptoms of seasonal allergies.

PHARMACOLOGY
Antihistamines antagonize H_1 receptors, opposing the effects of histamine.

INDICATIONS
Allergies, Insomnia (1st generation antihistamines), Motion Sickness (dimenhydrinate)

SIDE EFFECTS
Drowsiness (especially 1st generation antihistamines)

DRUG INTERACTIONS
Increased drowsiness when used with other drugs that suppress central nervous system activity (e.g., benzodiazepines, sedative-hypnotics, opioids, alcohol).

1ST GENERATION ANTIHISTAMINES
First-generation antihistamines (e.g., diphenhydramine, dimenhydrinate, doxylamine) readily cross the blood-brain barrier (BBB), antagonizing histamine receptors in the central nervous system and causing drowsiness. The link to sedation is so strong that diphenhydramine and doxylamine are marketed as over-the-counter sleep aids under the trade names ZzzQuil® and Unisom®, respectively.

PARADOXICAL EXCITATION
Antihistamines typically cause sedation; however, rarely patients may experience paradoxical excitation (e.g., insomnia, restlessness, tremor, hallucinations). Paradoxical excitation occurs most often in children.

2ND GENERATION ANTIHISTAMINES
Second-generation antihistamines (e.g., fexofenadine, loratadine, cetirizine) do not cross the BBB to a significant degree and, consequently, do not cause sedation. Nonetheless, some patients may still experience drowsiness, particularly with high doses. Second-generation antihistamines are marketed as "non-drowsy" and are generally more popular than their first-generation counterparts.

MAY CAUSE DROWSINESS

MUSCLE RELAXANTS
FOR MUSCLE SPASMS

BRAND NAME		GENERIC NAME
Lioresal®		Baclofen
Soma®	C-IV	Carisoprodol
Flexeril®		Cyclobenzaprine
Skelaxin®		Metaxalone
Robaxin®		Methocarbamol
Zanaflex®		Tizanidine

BACKGROUND
The nervous system mediates muscle contraction.

PHARMACOLOGY
Depress central nervous system activity, slowing the nerve signals that mediate muscle contraction.

INDICATIONS
Muscle Spasm, Pulled Muscle, Back Pain

SIDE EFFECTS
Drowsiness

MAY CAUSE DROWSINESS

DRUG INTERACTIONS
Increased drowsiness/sedation when combined with other drugs that suppress central nervous system activity (e.g., benzodiazepines, opioids, antihistamines, alcohol).

THE #1 SIDE EFFECT OF MUSCLE RELAXANTS: DROWSINESS
Patients should avoid driving or operating machinery until the effects are known.
Patients must not drink alcohol while taking these medications.

POTENTIAL FOR ABUSE
Muscle relaxants, even those that are not controlled substances, can be used by drug abusers to enhance the effect of other depressants, which is particularly dangerous, as it can lead to fatal respiratory depression.

HORMONE CONTRACEPTIVES
FOR PREGNANCY PREVENTION

BRAND NAME	GENERIC NAME	DOSAGE FORM/ PACKAGE CONTENTS
Ortho Cyclen®	Sprintec®	21 Active & 7 Inactive Tablets
Ortho Tri-Cyclen®	Tri-Sprintec®	21 Active & 7 Inactive Tablets
Yaz®	Gianvi®	24 Active & 4 Inactive Tablets
Loestrin® 24 Fe	Lomedia® 24 Fe	24 Active & 4 Iron Tablets
Ortho Evra®	Xulane®	Transdermal Patch
NuvaRing®	*	Intravaginal ring
Depo-Provera®	Medroxyprogesterone	Intramuscular Injection
Plan B One-Step®	Next Choice One Dose®	1 Emergency Contraceptive Tablet

*No generics available at the time of publication

BACKGROUND
Female hormones rise and fall in a pattern or "cycle" that promotes ovulation and implantation of an egg. During ovulation, the egg is released from the ovary. For an egg to be susceptible to fertilization by a sperm cell, ovulation must occur. Once fertilized, the egg needs to implant into the wall of the uterus to survive. If all three of these steps occur successfully–ovulation, fertilization, and implantation–then pregnancy occurs.

PHARMACOLOGY
Prevent ovulation or implantation of the egg.

INDICATIONS
Pregnancy Prevention

SIDE EFFECTS
Breast Tenderness, Nausea/Vomiting, Abdominal Pain, Emotional Changes, Blood Clots

DRUG INTERACTIONS
Smoking cigarettes increases the risk of blood clot formation. Antibiotics can reduce the effectiveness of hormone contraceptives.

KEEP IT SIMPLE
There are dozens of hormone contraceptive products. Most of them contain an estrogen and a progestin component. The names of the active ingredients can be long and complicated. Examples include norgestrel, norgestimate, levonorgestrel, desogestrel, norethindrone, and ethinyl estradiol. To reduce confusion, many generic manufacturers sell the generic versions under a brand name. For example, Ortho Cyclen® is generically available as Sprintec® & MonoNessa®, and Ortho Tri-Cyclen® is generically available as Tri-Sprintec® & TriNessa®. This is just the tip of the iceberg. Do not be overwhelmed by all of these names. The list above includes only the names of the most popular products along with details on how they are supplied/administered.

ALL HORMONE CONTRACEPTIVES ARE PREGNANCY CATEGORY X
NEVER TO BE USED DURING PREGNANCY

```
DO NOT USE IF
PREGNANT
```

ANTI-GOUT AGENTS FOR GOUT

BRAND NAME	GENERIC NAME
Zyloprim®	Allopurinol
Colcrys®	Colchicine
Uloric®	Febuxostat

BACKGROUND

Gout involves severe inflammation of one or more joints caused by high uric acid levels in the blood. Uric acid enters the blood after consuming certain foods and beverages, after cells in the body die. Certain drugs can also increase uric acid levels. When the concentration of uric acid in the blood gets too high, it crystallizes (i.e., turns to a solid), and the uric acid crystals deposit in joint spaces. The immune system attacks the uric acid crystals, thinking they are foreign invaders. The joints suffer collateral damage from the immune response, causing severe joint pain and inflammation (i.e., gout). The joint of the big toe is usually the first to be affected.

PHARMACOLOGY

Block the formation of uric acid (allopurinol, febuxostat) or prevent the immune system from attacking uric acid crystals (colchicine).

INDICATIONS

Gout

SIDE EFFECTS

Diarrhea, Nausea/Vomiting, Abdominal Cramps/Pain, Impaired White Blood Cell Formation/Development (colchicine)

DRUG INTERACTIONS

Many drugs can increase uric acid levels in the blood (e.g., aspirin and thiazide diuretics), which can work against uric acid lowering treatments.

GOUT AND NSAIDs

During a gout flare, practitioners often prescribe an NSAID to reduce joint pain and inflammation. Indocin® (Indomethacin) is a common choice among prescribers.

OPHTHALMIC PROSTAGLANDIN ANALOGS
FOR GLAUCOMA

BRAND NAME	GENERIC NAME
Lumigan®	Bimatoprost
Xalatan®	Latanoprost
Travatan®	Travoprost

Note: Notice that all of the generic names for prostaglandin analogs end in "-oprost."

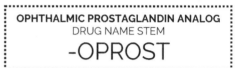

OPHTHALMIC PROSTAGLANDIN ANALOG
DRUG NAME STEM

-OPROST

BACKGROUND
The front of the eye is filled with a fluid called aqueous humor. Aqueous humor normally flows into and out of the eye in equal proportions, maintaining even pressure within the eye. In patients with glaucoma, there are problems, usually with the outflow of aqueous humor, that lead to elevated pressure within the eye. Over time, this high intraocular pressure damages the optic nerve. Minor vision loss is common, and if left untreated, the vision loss will eventually progress to complete blindness.

PHARMACOLOGY
Increase the outflow of aqueous humor, thus decreasing pressure within the eye. Prostaglandins are typically associated with inflammation, but in the eye, prostaglandins increase the outflow of aqueous humor.

INDICATIONS
Glaucoma

SIDE EFFECTS
Eyelash Growth, Dry Eye, Blurred Vision, Discoloration of the Iris, Inflammation of the Eye

DRUG INTERACTIONS
None

NOTES
The medications in this drug class are eye drops. Xalatan® (Latanoprost) should be stored in the refrigerator until opened. Once opened, Xalatan® can be stored at room temperature for up to 6 weeks, after which any remaining medication must be discarded. Lumigan® and Travatan® are stable at room temperature.

CAPITALIZING ON A SIDE EFFECT
Eyelash growth is a common side effect associated with the use of prostaglandin analogs. The side effect is so common that the drug manufacturer Allergen, Inc. reformulated bimatoprost to make another prescription-only product called Latisse®, designed specifically for cosmetic eyelash enhancement.

FOR THE EYE

OPHTHALMIC BETA-BLOCKERS FOR GLAUCOMA

BRAND NAME	GENERIC NAME
Timoptic®	Timolol
Betoptic S®	Betaxolol

Note: Notice that the generic names for beta-blockers end in "-olol."

BACKGROUND: Aqueous humor production also contributes to high intraocular pressure.

PHARMACOLOGY: Reduce the production of aqueous humor.

INDICATIONS: Glaucoma

SIDE EFFECTS: Bradycardia, Hypotension, Asthma and COPD Exacerbations

DRUG INTERACTIONS: May increase the risk of hypotension and bradycardia when used with other drugs that can lower blood pressure and reduce heart rate.

NOTES: We covered beta-blockers before in the high blood pressure section, but the beta-blockers listed here are supplied as eye drops explicitly created for the treatment of glaucoma.

FOR THE EYE

PROCEED TO THE NEXT SECTION TO MEMORIZE THE TOP 200 DRUGS

TOP 200 DRUGS

BRAND NAME	GENERIC NAME	PRIMARY INDICATION
Cleocin T®, Clindagel®	Clindamycin (Topical)	Acne
Retin-A®	Tretinoin (Topical)	Acne
Adderall®	Amphetamine/Dextroamphetamine *C-II*	ADHD
Vyvanse®	Lisdexamfetamine *C-II*	ADHD
Ritalin®	Methylphenidate *C-II*	ADHD
Concerta®	Methylphenidate (Extended Release) *C-II*	ADHD
Pataday®, Patanol®	Olopatadine (Ophthalmic)	Allergic Conjunctivitis
Flonase®	Fluticasone (Nasal)	Allergic Rhinitis
Zyrtec®	Cetirizine	Allergies
Allegra®	Fexofenadine	Allergies
Atarax®, Vistaril®	Hydroxyzine	Allergies, Anxiety
Claritin®	Loratadine	Allergies
Aricept®	Donepezil	Alzheimer's Disease
Namenda®	Memantine	Alzheimer's Disease
EpiPen®	Epinephrine	Anaphylaxis
Apresoline®	Hydralazine	Angina
Imdur®	Isosorbide Mononitrate	Angina
Nitrostat®	Nitroglycerin (Sublingual)	Angina
Hibiclens®	Chlorhexidine (Topical)	Antiseptic Cleanser
Xanax®	Alprazolam *C-IV*	Anxiety
Buspar®	Buspirone	Anxiety
Klonopin®	Clonazepam *C-IV*	Anxiety
Valium®	Diazepam *C-IV*	Anxiety
Ativan®	Lorazepam *C-IV*	Anxiety
AccuNeb®, ProAir®, Proventil®, Ventolin®	Albuterol (Inhaled)	Asthma
Qvar® RediHaler™	Beclomethasone (Inhaled)	Asthma
Symbicort®	Budesonide/Formoterol (Inhaled)	Asthma
Flovent®	Fluticasone (Inhaled)	Asthma
Advair®, AirDuo™	Fluticasone/Salmeterol (Inhaled)	Asthma
Breo Ellipta®	Fluticasone/Vilanterol (Inhaled)	Asthma
Singulair®	Montelukast	Asthma
Amoxil®	Amoxicillin	Bacterial Infections
Augmentin®	Amoxicillin/Clavulanate	Bacterial Infections
Zithromax®, Z-pak®	Azithromycin	Bacterial Infections
Omnicef®	Cefdinir	Bacterial Infections
Keflex®	Cephalexin	Bacterial Infections
Cipro®	Ciprofloxacin	Bacterial Infections
Cleocin®	Clindamycin	Bacterial Infections
Monodox®, Vibramycin®	Doxycycline	Bacterial Infections
Levaquin®	Levofloxacin	Bacterial Infections
Flagyl®	Metronidazole	Bacterial Infections
Bactroban®	Mupirocin (Topical)	Bacterial Infections
Pen-Vee K®	Penicillin V Potassium	Bacterial Infections
Bactrim®, Septra®	Sulfamethoxazole/Trimethoprim	Bacterial Infections
Yasmin®, Yaz®	Drospirenone/Ethinyl Estradiol	Birth Control
Seasonale®, Seasonique®	Levonorgestrel/Ethinyl Estradiol	Birth Control
Loestrin®, Microgestin®	Norethindrone/Ethinyl Estradiol	Birth Control
Ortho-Cyclen®, Sprintec®	Norgestimate/EthinylEstradiol	Birth Control
Eliquis®	Apixaban	Blood Clots

Ecotrin®	Aspirin	Blood Clots
Plavix®	Clopidogrel	Blood Clots
Xarelto®	Rivaroxaban	Blood Clots
Coumadin®, Jantoven®	Warfarin	Blood Clots
Cardura®	Doxazosin	BPH, Hypertension
Proscar®	Finasteride	BPH
Flomax®	Tamsulosin	BPH
Cordarone®, Pacerone®	Amiodarone	Cardiac Arrhythmias
Lanoxin®	Digoxin	Cardiac Arrhythmias
Restasis®	Cyclosporine (Ophthalmic)	Chronic Dry Eye
Colace®	Docusate	Constipation
Miralax®	Polyethylene Glycol 3350	Constipation
Combivent®, DuoNeb®	Ipratropium/Albuterol (Inhaled)	COPD
Spiriva®	Tiotropium (Inhaled)	COPD
Tessalon® Perles	Benzonatate	Cough
Cheratussin® AC, Virtussin® AC	Guaifenesin/Codeine *C-V*	Cough
Entocort® EC	Budesonide	Crohn's Disease
Elavil®	Amitriptyline	Depression
Wellbutrin®	Bupropion	Depression
Celexa®	Citalopram	Depression
Cymbalta®	Duloxetine	Depression
Lexapro®	Escitalopram	Depression
Prozac®	Fluoxetine	Depression
Remeron®	Mirtazapine	Depression
Pamelor®	Nortriptyline	Depression
Paxil®	Paroxetine	Depression
Zoloft®	Sertraline	Depression
Desyrel®	Trazodone	Depression, Insomnia
Effexor®	Venlafaxine	Depression
Amaryl®	Glimepiride	Diabetes
Glucotrol®	Glipizide	Diabetes
DiaBeta®, Micronase®	Glyburide	Diabetes
NovoLog®	Insulin Aspart	Diabetes
Levemir®	Insulin Detemir	Diabetes
Basaglar®, Lantus®, Toujeo®	Insulin Glargine	Diabetes
Humulin® N, Novolin® N	Insulin Isophane (NPH)	Diabetes
Humalog®	Insulin Lispro	Diabetes
Humulin® 70/30, Novolin® 70/30	Insulin NPH 70%/Regular Insulin 30%	Diabetes
Victoza®	Liraglutide	Diabetes
Glucophage®	Metformin	Diabetes
Actos®	Pioglitazone	Diabetes
Januvia®	Sitagliptin	Diabetes
Janumet®	Sitagliptin/Metformin	Diabetes
Carafate®	Sucralfate	Duodenal Ulcers
Diflucan®	Fluconazole	Fungal Infections
Nizoral®	Ketoconazole (Topical)	Fungal Infections
Mycostatin®, Nystop®	Nystatin (Topical)	Fungal Infections
Nexium®	Esomeprazole	GERD
Pepcid®	Famotidine	GERD
Prilosec®	Omeprazole	GERD
Protonix®	Pantoprazole	GERD
Zantac®	Ranitidine	GERD
Alphagan® P	Brimonidine (Ophthalmic)	Glaucoma

Cosopt®	Dorzolamide/Timolol (Ophthalmic)	Glaucoma
Xalatan®	Latanoprost (Ophthalmic)	Glaucoma
Timoptic®	Timolol (Ophthalmic)	Glaucoma
Zyloprim®	Allopurinol	Gout
Colcrys®	Colchicine	Gout
Lipitor®	Atorvastatin	High Cholesterol
Zetia®	Ezetimibe	High Cholesterol
Tricor®	Fenofibrate	High Cholesterol
Mevacor®	Lovastatin	High Cholesterol
Pravachol®	Pravastatin	High Cholesterol
Crestor®	Rosuvastatin	High Cholesterol
Zocor®	Simvastatin	High Cholesterol
Lopid®	Gemfibrozil	High Triglycerides
Lovaza®	Omega-3-Acid Ethyl Esters	High Triglycerides
Norvasc®	Amlodipine	Hypertension
Lotrel®	Amlodipine/Benazepril	Hypertension
Tenormin®	Atenolol	Hypertension
Lotensin®	Benazepril	Hypertension
Coreg®	Carvedilol	Hypertension
Hygroton®, Thalitone®	Chlorthalidone	Hypertension
Catapres®	Clonidine	Hypertension
Cardizem®, Tiazac®	Diltiazem	Hypertension
Vasotec®	Enalapril	Hypertension
Lasix®	Furosemide	Hypertension
Tenex®	Guanfacine	Hypertension, ADHD
Microzide®	Hydrochlorothiazide	Hypertension
Prinzide®, Zestoretic®	Hydrochlorothiazide/Lisinopril	Hypertension
Prinivil®, Zestril®	Lisinopril	Hypertension
Cozaar®	Losartan	Hypertension
Hyzaar®	Losartan/Hydrochlorothiazide	Hypertension
Toprol-XL®	Metoprolol Succinate (Extended Release)	Hypertension
Lopressor®	Metoprolol Tartrate	Hypertension
Bystolic®	Nebivolol	Hypertension
Nifediac®, Procardia®	Nifedipine	Hypertension
Inderal®	Propranolol	Hypertension
Altace®	Ramipril	Hypertension
Aldactone®	Spironolactone	Hypertension
Dyazide®, Maxzide®	Triamterene/Hydrochlorothiazide	Hypertension
Diovan®	Valsartan	Hypertension
Diovan HCT®	Valsartan/Hydrochlorothiazide	Hypertension
Calan®, Verelan®	Verapamil	Hypertension
K-Dur®, Klor-Con®	Potassium Chloride	Hypokalemia
Levoxyl®, Synthroid®	Levothyroxine	Hypothyroidism
Armour® Thyroid, Nature-Throid®, NP	Thyroid Desiccated	Hypothyroidism
Celebrex®	Celecoxib	Inflammation
Clobex®, Temovate®	Clobetasol (Topical)	Inflammation, Psoriasis
Voltaren®	Diclofenac	Inflammation
Cortizone-10®	Hydrocortisone (Topical)	Inflammation
Motrin®	Ibuprofen	Inflammation
Mobic®	Meloxicam	Inflammation
Trexall®	Methotrexate	Inflammation
Medrol®	Methylprednisolone	Inflammation
Naprosyn®	Naproxen	Inflammation

Orapred®	Prednisolone	Inflammation
Omnipred®, Pred Forte®	Prednisolone (Ophthalmic)	Inflammation
Deltasone®, Sterapred®	Prednisone	Inflammation
Kenalog®	Triamcinolone (Topical)	Inflammation
Restoril®	Temazepam *C-IV*	Insomnia
Ambien	Zolpidem *C-IV*	Insomnia
Bentyl®	Dicyclomine	Irritable Bowel Syndrome
Androgel®, Androderm®	Testosterone (Transdermal) *C-III*	Low Testosterone
Plaquenil®	Hydroxychloroquine	Malaria
Estrace®	Estradiol	Menopause
Provera®	Medroxyprogesterone	Menstrual Irregularities
Fioricet®	Butalbital/Acetaminophen/Caffeine	Migraines
Maxalt®	Rizatriptan	Migraines
Imitrex®	Sumatriptan	Migraines
Antivert®	Meclizine	Motion Sickness
Liorisal®	Baclofen	Muscle Spasms
Flexeril®	Cyclobenzaprine	Muscle Spasms
Robaxin®	Methocarbamol	Muscle Spasms
Zanaflex®	Tizanidine	Muscle Spasms
Zofran®	Ondansetron	Nausea/Vomiting
Phenergan®	Promethazine	Nausea/Vomiting
Neurontin®	Gabapentin	Nerve Pain, Seizures
Lyrica®	Pregabalin *C-V*	Nerve Pain, Seizures
Fosamax®	Alendronate	Osteoporosis
Ditropan®	Oxybutynin	Overactive Bladder
Tylenol®	Acetaminophen	Pain
Tylenol® #3	Codeine/Acetaminophen *C-III*	Pain
Hysingla™ ER, Zohydro™ ER	Hydrocodone (Extended Release) *C-II*	Pain
Lortab®, Norco®	Hydrocodone/Acetaminophen *C-II*	Pain
Lidoderm®	Lidocaine (Topical)	Pain
MS Contin®	Morphine Sulfate (Extended Release) *C-II*	Pain
Roxicodone®	Oxycodone *C-II*	Pain
OxyContin®	Oxycodone (Extended Release) *C-II*	Pain
Endocet®, Percocet®	Oxycodone/Acetaminophen *C-II*	Pain
Ultram®	Tramadol *C-IV*	Pain
Requip®	Ropinirole	Parkinson's Disease
Abilify®	Aripiprazole	Psychiatric Disorders
Seroquel®	Quetiapine	Psychiatric Disorders
Risperdal®	Risperidone	Psychiatric Disorders
Depakote®	Divalproex	Seizures
Lamictal®	Lamotrigine	Seizures
Keppra®	Levetiracetam	Seizures
Topamax®	Topiramate	Seizures
Zyban®	Bupropion	Smoking Cessation
Macrobid®, Macrodantin®	Nitrofurantoin	Urinary Tract Infections
Zovirax®	Acyclovir	Viral Infections
Tamiflu®	Oseltamivir	Viral Infections (Influenza)
Valtrex®	Valacyclovir	Viral Infections
Adipex-P®	Phentermine *C-IV*	Weight Loss

Please note that the current list of the top 200 drugs contains 204 items due to the repeated appearance of four active ingredients (metoprolol, bupropion, methylphenidate, and oxycodone).

TOP 50 OTC DRUGS

Over the counter (OTC) medications are drugs that are available to patients without a prescription for self-treatment of minor medical conditions. The Top 50 OTC Drugs below are categorized by drug class.

OTC PAIN MEDICATIONS

BRAND NAME	GENERIC NAME	DRUG CLASS
Tylenol®	Acetaminophen	Analgesic/Antipyretic
Advil®, Motrin®	Ibuprofen	Non-Steroidal Anti-inflammatory Drug
Aleve®	Naproxen	Non-Steroidal Anti-inflammatory Drug
Ecotrin®	Aspirin	Non-Steroidal Anti-inflammatory Drug
Excedrin® Migraine	Acetaminophen/Aspirin/Caffeine	Combination Analgesic for Migraines
Azo®	Phenazopyridine	Urinary Analgesic*

*Azo® (Phenazopyridine) is only effective for urinary pain/burning.

OTC ANTACIDS

BRAND NAME	GENERIC NAME	DRUG CLASS
Alka-Seltzer®	Citric Acid/Sodium Bicarbonate	Antacid
Gaviscon®	Aluminum Hydroxide/Magnesium Carbonate	Antacid
Maalox®	Aluminum Hydroxide/Magnesium Hydroxide/Simethicone	Antacid
Mylanta®	Aluminum Hydroxide/Magnesium Hydroxide/Simethicone	Antacid
Tums®	Calcium Carbonate	Antacid
Pepcid®	Famotidine	H2 Blocker
Tagamet®	Cimetidine	H2 Blocker
Zantac®	Ranitidine	H2 Blocker
Nexium®	Esomeprazole	Proton Pump Inhibitor
Prevacid®	Lansoprazole	Proton Pump Inhibitor
Prilosec OTC®	Omeprazole	Proton Pump Inhibitor

*Most antacids are effective for heartburn, indigestion, nausea, and upset stomach. Antacids that contain aluminum or calcium are preferred for patients with diarrhea, and antacids with simethicone are good for reducing gas and bloating.

OTC LAXATIVES

BRAND NAME	GENERIC NAME	DRUG CLASS
Metamucil®	Psyllium Fiber	Fiber Laxative
Citrate of Magnesium	Magnesium Citrate	Osmotic Laxative
Milk of Magnesia®	Magnesium Hydroxide	Osmotic Laxative
Miralax®	Polyethylene Glycol (PEG) 3350	Osmotic Laxative
Dulcolax®	Bisacodyl	Stimulant Laxative
Senokot®	Sennosides	Stimulant Laxative
Colace®	Docusate	Stool Softener
Senokot-S®	Docusate/Sennosides	Stool Softener/Stimulant Laxative

*Laxatives are effective for constipation.

OTC GASTROINTESTINAL MEDICATIONS

BRAND NAME	GENERIC NAME	DRUG CLASS
Imodium®	Loperamide	Antidiarrheal
Pepto-Bismol®	Bismuth Subsalicylate	Antidiarrheal*
Emetrol®	Dextrose/Fructose/Phosphoric Acid	Antiemetic
Gas-X®	Simethicone	Aniflatulent

*Pepto-Bismol® is also used to treat heartburn, nausea, upset stomach, and H. pylori infections.

OTC COUGH & COLD MEDICATIONS

BRAND NAME	GENERIC NAME	DRUG CLASS
Chloraseptic® Sore Throat Spray	Phenol (Oropharyngeal)	Anesthetic/Analgesic
Delsym®	Dextromethorphan	Cough Suppressant
Sudafed®	Pseudoephedrine	Decongestant
Robitussin®	Guaifenesin	Expectorant
Afrin® Nasal Spray	Oxymetazoline	Nasal Decongestant
Neo-Synephrine® Nasal Spray	Phenylephrine	Nasal Decongestant

OTC ALLERGY MEDICATIONS

BRAND NAME	GENERIC NAME	DRUG CLASS
Benadryl®	Diphenhydramine	Antihistamine (1st Generation)
Chlor-Trimeton®	Chlorpheniramine	Antihistamine (1st Generation)
Allegra®	Fexofenadine	Antihistamine (2nd Generation)
Claritin®, Alavert®	Loratadine	Antihistamine (2nd Generation)
Zaditor®, Alaway® Eye Drops	Ketotifen	Antihistamine (2nd Generation)
Zyrtec®	Cetirizine	Antihistamine (2nd Generation)
Flonase® Nasal Spray	Fluticasone	Corticosteroid
Nasacort® Nasal Spray	Triamcinolone	Corticosteroid

OTC CREAMS, OINTMENTS, AND GELS

BRAND NAME	GENERIC NAME	DRUG CLASS
Solarcaine®	Lidocaine	Anesthetic
Neosporin®	Bacitracin/Neomycin/Polymyxin-B	Antibiotic
Lamisil®	Terbinafine	Antifungal
Lamisil® AF	Tolnaftate	Antifungal
Lotrimin®	Clotrimazole	Antifungal
Monistat® Vaginal Cream	Miconazole	Antifungal
Zeasorb®	Miconazole	Antifungal

*OTC antifungals are generally effective for minor topical fungal infections
(e.g., jock itch, athlete's foot, and ringworm).

VITAMINS

For people without vitamin deficiencies, the best way to obtain vitamins is through a well-balanced diet of wholesome foods. There are two categories of vitamins: fat-soluble and water-soluble. Fat-soluble vitamins include vitamin A, D, E, and K. All other vitamins are water-soluble (all of the B vitamins and vitamin C). Excessive doses of fat-soluble vitamins (A, D, E, and K) accumulate in fat tissue over time, potentially leading to toxicity/adverse health effects. Excessive doses of water-soluble vitamins quickly exit the body by way of the urine and generally cause fewer problems. Keep in mind that, while rare, excessive doses of certain water-soluble vitamins can still produce adverse effects; for example, excessive doses of vitamin C can cause diarrhea.

Vitamin A (Retinol)
Uses: Needed for low-light vision.
Recommended adult dose: 2,000 – 3,000 IU/day
Max dose: 10,000 IU/day; excessive doses during pregnancy can cause birth defects.
Notes: When beta-carotene is consumed, from carrots and sweet potatoes, for instance, it is converted to vitamin A inside the body.

Vitamin B1 (Thiamine)
Uses: Needed for metabolism of carbohydrates.
Recommended adult dose: 1 – 1.5 mg/day (10 mg/day for cataract prevention)
Max dose: None established.

Vitamin B2 (Riboflavin)
Uses: Needed for metabolism of fats, proteins, and carbohydrates.
Recommended adult dose: 1 mg/day
Max dose: None established.

Vitamin B3 (Niacin)
Uses: Lowers cholesterol and triglycerides.
Recommended adult dose: 14 – 18 mg/day
Max dose: 35 mg/day; high doses cause flushing.
Notes: Flushing can be prevented by taking an NSAID (e.g., aspirin) with the niacin.

Vitamin B5 (Pantothenic Acid)
Uses: Needed for metabolism of nutrients and synthesis of certain enzymes.
Recommended adult dose: 5 mg/day
Max Dose: None established; excessive doses can cause diarrhea.

Vitamin B6 (Pyridoxine)
Uses: Needed for metabolism, immune function, and fetal brain development.
Recommended adult dose: 1.5 mg/day
Max dose: 100 mg for adults; excessive doses can cause severe nerve damage.

Vitamin B7 (Biotin)
Uses: Needed for metabolism of nutrients. Commonly used to help strengthen nails and hair.
Recommended adult dose: 30 mcg/day
Max dose: None established.

Vitamin B9 (Folic Acid)
Uses: Needed for cell development; routinely used by women during pregnancy to prevent fetal neural tube defects.
Recommended adult dose: 400 mcg/day (600 mcg/day for pregnant women)
Max dose: 1,000 mcg/day (higher doses may be used for certain conditions).

Vitamin B12 (Cobalamin)
Uses: Needed for DNA and red blood cell production.
Recommended adult dose: ~ 2.4 mcg/day
Max dose: None established (high doses have not demonstrated harm).
Notes: A protein in the stomach called "intrinsic factor" is needed to absorb vitamin B12. Patients deficient in this protein develop vitamin B12 deficiency (a condition known as "pernicious anemia"). Like other types of anemia, this condition is characterized by a low red blood cell count. The diabetes drug Glucophage® (metformin) is notorious for interfering with the body's ability to absorb vitamin B12.

Vitamin C (Ascorbic Acid)
Uses: Needed for its antioxidant properties to protect cells from free radical damage; the body also uses vitamin C in collagen production, which is needed for wound healing.
Recommended adult dose: 75 – 100 mg/day
Max dose: 2,000 mg/day; excessive doses can cause diarrhea and iron overload.
Notes: Vitamin C deficiency causes scurvy. Taking vitamin C with an iron supplement will increase the intestinal absorption of iron.

Vitamin D (Ergocalciferol (D2), Cholecalciferol (D3))
Uses: Needed for nerve function, immune function, and most notably for the absorption of dietary calcium.
Recommended adult dose: 400 – 800 IU/day
Max dose: 4,000 IU/day; excessive doses can cause kidney damage and/or high calcium levels, leading to cardiac arrhythmias.
Notes: Vitamin D deficiency causes rickets in children and osteomalacia in adults, which are conditions characterized by softening/weakening of the bones. *Xenical® (orlistat)* and *Alli® (orlistat)* are weight-loss drugs that work by reducing the intestinal absorption of fats. Because they block fat absorption, these drugs can lead to a deficiency in fat-soluble vitamins (A, D, E, and K), including vitamin D.

Vitamin E (Alpha-Tocopherol and seven other related compounds)
Uses: Needed for its antioxidant properties to protect cells from free radical damage; the body also needs vitamin E for immune function and cardiovascular health.
Recommended adult dose: 22 IU/day
Max dose: 1,100 – 1,500 IU/day; excessive doses can cause bleeding.
Notes: Vitamin E deficiency is rare but can cause nerve damage, muscle damage, and a weakened immune system. The risk of experiencing bleeding while taking vitamin E is especially high for patients on antiplatelet or anticoagulant medications like *aspirin, clopidogrel, warfarin,* and *heparin*.

A NOTE ABOUT ANTIOXIDANTS
Antioxidants tend to interfere with cancer chemotherapy and radiation therapy, thus reducing the effectiveness of these treatments. Why? Because antioxidants protect cells (including cancer cells) from free radicals, and often free radicals (such as radiation) are used as a form of therapy to kill cancer cells.

Vitamin K (Phytonadione)
Uses: Essential for blood clot formation; sometimes used topically to treat rosacea, stretch marks, scars, and burns; most notably used orally or by injection to reverse the effects of warfarin.
Recommended dose: 90 – 120 mcg/day
Max dose: None established.
Notes: Consumption of vitamin K-containing foods should be consistent for patients taking warfarin. If a patient ingests more than their usual amount of vitamin K while using warfarin, he/she is at a higher risk for blood clots. If a patient consumes less than their usual amount of vitamin K while using warfarin, he/she is at a higher risk for bleeding.

TOP 30 HERBAL SUPPLEMENTS

Herbal supplements rarely have conclusive data to show that they are safe and effective in treating medical conditions. For this reason, pharmacists typically do not recommend the use of herbal supplements. Nonetheless, herbal supplements can be appropriate in some cases, and some patients choose to make use of these products. Below is a list of the Top 30 Herbal Supplements and their primary uses.

Aloe: Heal burns/wounds topically and promote digestive health when ingested

Biotin: Strengthen hair and nails

Black Cohosh: Alleviate symptoms of menopause

Cinnamon: Decrease blood sugar in patients with diabetes

Coenzyme Q-10: Promote cardiovascular health

Echinacea: Boost the immune system

Evening Primrose Oil: Alleviate symptoms of menopause

Feverfew: Alleviate migraine headaches

Fish Oil: Promote cardiovascular health and decrease blood triglyceride levels

Flaxseed Oil: Reduce inflammation and lower blood cholesterol levels

Folic Acid: Prevent fetal neural tube defects (taken before & during pregnancy)

Garlic: Decrease blood pressure

Ginger: Reduce nausea

Gingko: Improve memory and increase blood circulation

Glucosamine & Chondroitin: Alleviate osteoarthritis pain

Green Tea: Increase metabolism; cancer prevention (antioxidant properties)

Hoodia: Promote weight-loss

Kava Kava: Reduce symptoms of anxiety

Melatonin: Promote sleep; may be used in the treatment of insomnia

Milk Thistle: Promote liver health

Peppermint: Alleviate heartburn and upset stomach

Probiotics: Promote digestive health

Red Yeast Rice: Lower blood cholesterol levels

St. John's Wort: Improve depression (this supplement has *many* drug interactions)

SAM-e: Stabilize mood

Saw Palmetto: Reduce prostate size in patients with BPH

Senna: Stimulate bowel movements

Valerian: Promote sleep and reduce symptoms of anxiety

Witch Hazel: Treat various skin conditions

Yohimbe: Treat erectile dysfunction (this supplement can raise blood pressure)

COMMON DRUG INTERACTIONS

DRUG-DRUG INTERACTIONS

Warfarin and NSAIDs*

> Warfarin is an anticoagulant used to prevent or treat blood clots. A major side effect of warfarin is bleeding. NSAIDs are notorious for damaging the lining of the stomach, which has the potential to lead to a gastrointestinal bleed. When warfarin and NSAIDs are used together, the risk of a life-threatening GI bleed increases significantly. NSAIDs also have some "anti-platelet" (blood-thinning) effect, which further increases bleed risk. *Some examples of generic NSAIDs include Ibuprofen, Naproxen, Aspirin, Meloxicam, Indomethacin, and Diclofenac.

Warfarin and Antibiotics

> Antibiotics increase the bleeding risk associated with warfarin. The reason for this is explained below.

> ### How Warfarin Works
> The body uses Vitamin K to activate the "vitamin K-dependent clotting factors" (factors 2, 7, 9, and 10). Once vitamin K is used to activate a clotting factor, it is deactivated, rendered incapable of activating more clotting factors unless it is reactivated by the enzyme "Vitamin K Epoxide Reductase Complex 1" (VKORC1). Warfarin inhibits VKORC1, thus preventing activation of vitamin K-dependent clotting factors. In simpler terms, warfarin reduces blood clotting by keeping vitamin K in its deactivated form. Since vitamin K is deactivated, it cannot activate certain clotting factors.

> ### Why Antibiotics Interact with Warfarin
> Vitamin K enters the body from two sources: the diet (e.g., green leafy vegetables, mayonnaise) and intestinal flora (healthy bacteria that reside in the intestine). Intestinal flora produces vitamin K, which gets absorbed into the bloodstream. When antibiotics are introduced into the body, some of the intestinal flora is killed. Since there are fewer bacteria producing vitamin K in the intestine, less vitamin K enters the bloodstream from that source, which amplifies warfarin's effect, potentially leading to over-anticoagulation and bleeding.

Oral Contraceptives and Antibiotics

> Antibiotics can decrease the effect of oral contraceptives, which increases the likelihood of contraceptive failure and increases risk of pregnancy. The prevailing theory behind this interaction is reduced enterohepatic circulation of estrogen caused by antibiotic-induced reduction of intestinal flora.

> ### Enterohepatic Circulation of Estrogen
> Some estrogen is eliminated by excretion into the bile where is carried out of the body during defecation. Some of the estrogen that goes into the bile gets hydrolyzed by intestinal flora and subsequently reabsorbed into the blood where it is given another opportunity to exert its pharmacologic effect. Since antibiotics kill intestinal flora, less estrogen gets hydrolyzed and reabsorbed (i.e., the effect of estrogen is reduced).

Vasodilators/Nitrates and PDE-5 Inhibitors

> Both of these drugs dilate blood vessels. When taken together, blood pressure can drop to a dangerously low level. PDE-5 inhibitors include Viagra® (sildenafil), Levitra® (vardenafil), and Cialis® (tadalafil).

Lithium and Diuretics

Lithium is used as a mood stabilizer in psychiatric disorders, and it can also be used to treat/prevent migraine headaches. Lithium is considered to be a "narrow therapeutic index drug," which means that there is less than a 2-fold difference between the median lethal dose and the median effective dose, or there is less than a 2-fold difference between the minimum toxic concentration and the minimum effective concentration. In other words, if the concentration of the drug in the blood gets too high, this therapeutic agent becomes a deadly toxin. The kidneys, which act as a filtration system for the blood, take lithium from the blood so it can leave the body in the urine. Diuretics work by causing the kidneys to transfer more than normal amounts of sodium and water from the blood into the urine. When more sodium is filtered out of the blood by the kidneys, a higher-than-normal amount of lithium is absorbed from the urine back into the blood. As a result, when taking diuretics while on lithium therapy, the concentration of lithium in the blood increases. This can lead to lithium toxicity and, in severe cases, death.

DRUG-NUTRIENT INTERACTIONS

HMG-CoA Reductase Inhibitors (Statins) and Grapefruit Juice

Grapefruit juice contains a group of substances chemically known as furanocoumarins, which irreversibly inhibit CYP3A4, a key enzyme involved in the metabolism of some statins. When taken together, statin levels in the blood increase, heightening the risk of statin-induced rhabdomyolysis.

Levodopa and Protein

Levodopa is used to treat symptoms of Parkinson's Disease. Dietary protein (e.g., from meat, nuts, and dairy products) interferes with the intestinal absorption of levodopa. Proteins also interfere with levodopa crossing the blood-brain barrier, which levodopa must cross to reach its site of action. As a result, when levodopa is taken with a high protein meal, less levodopa reaches the site of action (the brain).

Warfarin and Foods High in Vitamin K*

Since warfarin interferes with the activity of vitamin K, warfarin's effect can be reduced if dietary vitamin K intake increases. As a general rule, patients on warfarin should not avoid vitamin K but should make an effort to be consistent in how much vitamin K they consume each day. *Foods high in vitamin K include spinach, kale, collard greens, turnip greens, broccoli, Brussels sprouts, mayonnaise, green tea, and canola oil.

Note: Some multivitamins contain vitamin K.

DRUG-DISEASE INTERACTIONS

Decongestants* and Hypertension

When sinus blood vessels are swollen, they leak fluid and cause sinus congestion. Decongestants provide relief by constricting blood vessels. The blood vessels that are constricted by decongestants are not limited to those located in the sinus passages. Decongestants constrict blood vessels throughout the body, increasing blood pressure. In severe cases, use of a decongestant by an individual with hypertension could result in a cardiovascular event (e.g., stroke, aneurysm). *Decongestants include Sudafed® (pseudoephedrine) and Sudafed® PE (phenylephrine).

Aspirin and Peptic Ulcer Disease

Aspirin has an antiplatelet effect, which predisposes patients to bleeding. Aspirin is also notorious for causing damage to the lining of the stomach. A patient with peptic ulcer disease will have one or more lesions in the lining of their stomach, which can be irritated by aspirin, potentially leading to a gastrointestinal bleed.

DRUG NAME STEMS

When trying to determine the function of a drug, sometimes you will find a clue in the drug name itself. These clues are "drug name stems" and, when present, they usually appear as a suffix in the generic name of a drug. Below are some examples:

-afil = phosphodiesterase 5 (PDE–5) inhibitor (e.g., tadalafil, sildenafil, vardenafil) for erectile dysfunction.

-azepam or **–azolam** = benzodiazepine (e.g., alprazolam, clonazepam, oxazepam, diazepam) for anxiety and/or insomnia.

-azole = antifungal (e.g., clotrimazole, ketoconazole) for fungal infections.

-barbital = barbiturate or barbiturate derivative (e.g., phenobarbital, pentobarbital, secobarbital, amobarbital) for seizures.

ceph- or **cef-** = cephalosporin antibiotic (e.g., cephalexin, cefazolin, ceftriaxone, ceftazidime, cefdinir) for bacterial infections.

-dronate = bisphosphonate (e.g., ibandronate, alendronate, risedronate) for osteoporosis.

-floxacin = fluoroquinolone antibiotic (e.g., ciprofloxacin, moxifloxacin, levofloxacin) for bacterial infections.

-gliptin = dipeptidyl peptidase 4 (DPP-4) inhibitor (e.g., saxagliptin, sitagliptin, linagliptin) for type II diabetes.

-icillin = penicillin antibiotic (e.g., penicillin, amoxicillin, ampicillin, methicillin) for bacterial infections.

-olol = beta-blocker (e.g., metoprolol, atenolol, propranolol, bisoprolol) for hypertension and arrhythmias.

-oprost = prostaglandin analog (e.g., latanoprost) for glaucoma.

-osin = alpha-adrenergic receptor blocker (α-blocker) (e.g., doxazosin, terazosin, prazosin, tamsulosin) for high blood pressure and/or benign prostatic hyperplasia (BPH).

-prazole = proton pump inhibitor (PPI) (e.g., omeprazole, lansoprazole, pantoprazole, rabeprazole) for GERD.

-pril = angiotensin converting enzyme inhibitor (ACEI) (e.g., lisinopril, benazepril) used to lower blood pressure.

-sartan = angiotensin receptor blocker (ARB) (e.g., valsartan, losartan, olmesartan) for hypertension.

-setron = 5-HT$_3$ (serotonin) antagonist (e.g., ondansetron, palonosetron, granisetron) for nausea and vomiting.

-sone or **-solone** = corticosteroid (e.g., dexamethasone, prednisone, methylprednisolone) for inflammation.

-statin = HMG-CoA reductase inhibitor (e.g., atorvastatin, simvastatin, lovastatin, pravastatin) for high cholesterol.

-tidine = H2 receptor blockers (e.g., ranitidine, famotidine, cimetidine) for GERD.

-triptan = serotonin agonist (5-HT agonist) (e.g., sumatriptan, zolmitriptan, naratriptan, eletriptan) for migraine headaches.

-vir = antiviral (e.g., ritonavir, lopinavir, acyclovir, valacyclovir) for viral infections like shingles, genital herpes, and HIV/AIDS.

DOSAGE FORMS

Drug products are available in a variety of dosage forms. The dosage form is essentially the vehicle that delivers the drug to the site of action or the site of absorption. For a drug that acts locally, such as topical creams for conditions of the skin or ophthalmic drops for conditions of the eye, the manufacturer uses a dosage form that delivers the drug directly to the site of action. For drugs that exert their effect at some location inside the body, the manufacturer uses a dosage form that delivers the drug to a site of absorption (usually the gastrointestinal tract) where the drug enters the bloodstream. Manufacturers also select dosage forms based on answers to the following types of questions:

Does the drug dissolve in a liquid medium?
- Yes: Liquid Dosage Form
- No: Solid Dosage Form or Liquid Suspension

Does the drug dissolve better in water, alcohol, or oil?
- Water: Suspension or Syrup
- Alcohol: Elixir or Tincture
- Oil: Emulsion

Does the drug irritate the lining of the stomach?
- Yes: Enteric-Coated Tablet or Delayed-Release Tablet or Capsule
- No: Regular Tablet or Capsule

Do we want the patient to be able to break the doses into fractions?
- Yes: Scored Tablet
- No: Regular Tablet

From what location do we want the drug to be absorbed?
- The Stomach and Intestines: Tablet, Capsule, Suspension, or Solution
- The Intestines Only: Enteric-Coated Tablet, Delayed-Release Tablet or Capsule
- The Mouth: Sublingual Tablet or Buccal Lozenge
- The Skin: Transdermal Patch
- The Rectum: Rectal Suppository

For locally acting drugs, where will the patient apply the medication?
- The Skin: Cream, Ointment, Gel, or Lotion
- The Nose: Nasal Spray
- The Eye: Ophthalmic Drop
- The Ear: Otic Drop
- The Lungs: Inhaler or Nebulizer Solution

NOTE: Because of the inactive ingredients present in otic preparations, they cannot be used in the eye; however, ophthalmic preparations can be used in the ear if necessary.

LIQUID DOSAGE FORMS

Solution – A solute and a solvent; the solute molecules dissolve to form a homogeneous, single-phase mixture with the solvent.
General Example: Saltwater
Pharmaceutical Example: The liquid in an EpiPen® (epinephrine solution for injection)

Syrup – Highly concentrated water-based sugar solutions.
General Example: Maple syrup
Pharmaceutical Example: Ipecac syrup

Elixir – Solutions containing water, alcohol, and sweetener.
General Example: certain mixed alcoholic drinks (alcohol, ice/water, and sugar)
Pharmaceutical Example: Lortab® Elixir (hydrocodone/acetaminophen oral solution)

Tincture – Usually alcoholic extracts of crude materials. Alcohol content generally ranges from 15 – 80% for tinctures.
General Example: Tincture of iodine
Pharmaceutical Example: Paregoric® (camphorated tincture of opium)

> CONTAINS ALCOHOL

Suspension – A mixture of particles dispersed in a fluid medium; the particles do not dissolve, so the mixture is two-phase. *
General Example: Sand in water
Pharmaceutical Example: Mycostatin® (nystatin oral suspension)

Emulsion – A mixture in which one liquid is suspended in another.
General Example: Oil in water
Pharmaceutical Example: Restasis® (cyclosporine ophthalmic emulsion)

> SHAKE WELL

*Two-phase mixtures (i.e. suspensions and emulsions) must be shaken prior to dispensing and before each dose to ensure the medication is evenly distributed throughout the liquid medium. To alert the patient to this fact, you should place a "shake well" auxiliary label on the bottle of any suspension or emulsion you dispense. To understand the importance of this concept, look at the illustration below. Imagine that the drug is represented by the gray phase. If the patient does not "shake well," then the patient will receive less drug in the first few doses and much more drug in the last few doses.

Illustration: Why Suspensions & Emulsions Must Be Shaken

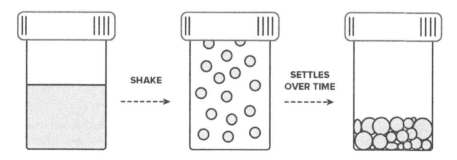

SOLID DOSAGE FORMS

Tablet
A powdery mixture of an active pharmaceutical ingredient and excipients (inert/inactive ingredients, such as fillers, binders, and colorants) pressed into a disc or other small shape. Tablets are the most popular dosage form.

Scored Tablet
Certain tablets should never be broken. For instance, most extended release tablets and capsules *must* be swallowed whole because splitting them can destroy the slow release mechanism and cause an overdose. On the other hand, some tablets are designed by the manufacturer with an indentation (i.e., they are "scored") to make it easy for the patient to divide the tablet into fractions. Below is an illustration of two scored tablets. On the left, we see a tablet that is scored into equal quarters. On the right, we see a tablet that is scored into equal halves. The illustration shows the top view of the tablet and the side view (rotated 90 degrees on the dashed-line axis) to illustrate the indentation better.

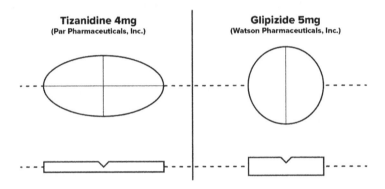

Tizanidine 4mg
(Par Pharmaceuticals, Inc.)

Glipizide 5mg
(Watson Pharmaceuticals, Inc.)

Enteric-Coated (EC) Tablet
An enteric coating is composed of special material that will not dissolve in the acidic environment of the stomach but will dissolve in the more neutral environment of the small intestines. As a result, when enteric-coated tablets are ingested, they do not dissolve until after they pass through the stomach and enter the small intestine. Manufacturers apply this coating for medications that would otherwise irritate or damage the lining of the stomach. An example is enteric-coated aspirin.

TAKE WHOLE DO NOT CRUSH OR CHEW

Sublingual (SL) Tablet
Sublingual tablets dissolve under the tongue, delivering medication across the tissue beneath the tongue, directly into the bloodstream. By entering the bloodstream directly, the drug can exert its pharmacologic effect much faster. A great example is the nitroglycerin sublingual tablet.

DISSOLVE UNDER TONGUE, DO NOT SWALLOW WHOLE

Orally Disintegrating Tablet (ODT)
Orally disintegrating tablets dissolve in the saliva. They are especially useful for patients that experience difficulty or pain when swallowing. For example, let's say a patient has experienced severe nausea and vomiting. While vomiting, acid from the stomach has damaged the lining of the patient's esophagus, making it painful to swallow. The anti-nausea medication ondansetron is available as an ODT for situations such as this.

DISSOLVE IN MOUTH DO NOT SWALLOW WHOLE

Capsule

Capsules are composed of two parts: the shell (usually made of hard gelatin) and the contents (drug powder, pellets, or tiny tablets). Many drugs are available in capsule form. Capsules are one of the most popular dosage forms, second only to tablets.

Soft Gelatin Capsule

Also commonly referred to as "gel caps" or "soft gels," this rendition of the capsule is usually yellow or amber and has a relatively transparent shell with liquid contents. Lovaza® and Tessalon® Perles are good examples.

Caplet

Capsule-shaped tablets. Tylenol® Extra Strength and Valtrex® are good examples.

Lozenge

Medicated candies designed to dissolve slowly – and thus release medication slowly – within the oral cavity. A good example is the Cepacol® Sore Throat Lozenge, which delivers benzocaine and menthol directly to the throat area. Clotrimazole is another example, which is available as a "tablet lozenge" for the treatment of oral thrush. Tablet lozenges have the appearance of a tablet, usually white and chalky, but they dissolve in the mouth like a traditional candy lozenge.

Troche

Technically, these are compressed lozenges, but many healthcare professionals use the terms "lozenge" and "troche" interchangeably.

MODIFIED RELEASE vs. IMMEDIATE RELEASE

Certain medications are available in a standard immediate release version and a special modified-release version. The immediate release versions dissolve quickly. Since immediate release is the default/standard version of a medication, the FDA does not require the drug package label to specify "immediate release." Otherwise, a vast majority of medications would have this term printed on their labels. Another term for immediate release is "regular release."

On the other hand, modified-release formulations (i.e., extended release and delayed-release) have a mechanism that controls the release of medication from the dosage form. Modified release is a broad term that encompasses two possible medication release mechanisms. #1 The "delayed release" mechanism (abbreviated "DR"), which is equivalent to an enteric coating. This mechanism delays the release of the medication until the dosage form (i.e. tablet, capsule, or particulate matter in a liquid suspension) passes through the stomach and enters the small intestine. #2 The "extended release" mechanism (abbreviated "ER"), which works by slowing the rate of medication release from a dosage form. Several processes have been designed to achieve the extended release effect, and, for that reason, there are several names and abbreviations that all essentially mean, "extended release." See the chart below for some common examples.

Modified Release Mechanism	Abbreviation(s)	Example(s)
Controlled Delivery	CD	Metadate CD®
Controlled Release	CR	Paxil CR®, Ambien CR®
Extended Release	ER, XL, XR	Depakote® ER, Toprol-XL®, Quillivant XR®
Long Acting	LA	Detrol® LA
Sustained Release	SR	Wellbutrin SR®

Note: According to the United States Pharmacopoeia (USP), delayed-release is synonymous with enteric-coated. All other modified-release dosage forms (CD, CR, LA, ER, XL, XR, and SR) employ some version of a slow release mechanism.

```
SWALLOW WHOLE
DO NOT CRUSH OR CHEW
```

SEMI-SOLID DOSAGE FORMS

Semi-solid dosage forms include ointments, creams, gels, and pastes. These dosage forms are most commonly used for topical applications (on the skin), but they can also be formulated for application to other sites. Examples include erythromycin ophthalmic ointment, Premarin® vaginal cream, Ayr® saline nasal gel, Proctozone-HC rectal ointment, and Prevident® 5000 Plus toothpaste.

Ointments
Ointments are mixtures of medication in a base of petroleum jelly or something similar to petroleum jelly. Ointments often have a greasy texture and tend to sit on top of the skin. This creates a moisture barrier that can be beneficial for dry skin. Because ointments sit on top of the skin, they deliver medication slower and over a longer period of time compared to other topical dosage forms. An example is Neosporin®.

Creams
Creams are typically medicated emulsions of oil-in-water that are easy to wash off. Compared to ointments, creams are lighter, less sticky, and less greasy. Creams tend to rub into the skin rather than sit on top as ointments do. Because they rub into the skin, creams release medication faster than ointments. An example is Lotrimin® AF cream.

Gels
Gels are mixtures of medication in a water-based medium. A gelling agent gives the water base a jelly-like consistency. Examples include Finacea® topical gel and Diastat® rectal gel.

Pastes
Pastes are thicker and stiffer than the other semi-solid dosage forms. Because of their thickness, they tend to penetrate the skin poorly, but they are effective skin protectants. The most common place we see paste dosage forms is dental preparations. An example is Biotene® dry mouth toothpaste.

LOTIONS

Lotions
Lotions are typically oil-in-water emulsions in a water-based medium. If you recall, creams are also oil-in-water emulsions. The same characteristics that apply to creams also apply to lotions. For example, they both tend to be less greasy and less sticky compared to ointments. The big difference between a cream and a lotion is the integration of a water-based medium, making lotions thinner and easier to spread. Because lotions are not as thick and stiff as ointments, creams, gels, and pastes, we do not consider them "semi-solids."

INHALATION SOLUTIONS, AEROSOLS, AND POWDERS

There are three major types of inhalable dosage forms: nebulizer solutions, metered dose inhalers, and dry powder inhalers. All of these dosage forms involve the administration of drug products by oral inhalation.

Nebulizer Solutions
Medicated solutions that are vaporized via air pressure generated by a machine called a nebulizer. Examples include AccuNeb®, DouNeb®, and Atrovent®.

Metered Dose Inhalers (MDIs)
Handheld devices that propel aerosolized drug particles when actuated. Chlorofluorocarbons (CFCs) were once the propellant of choice for MDIs, but the government outlawed the use of CFCs since they degrade ozone. The new propellant of choice used by manufacturers is the hydrofluoroalkanes (HFAs). Examples include Ventolin® HFA, ProAir® HFA, and Proventil® HFA.

Dry Powder Inhalers
A unique type of inhaler that does not contain propellants. Instead, the medication is supplied as a powder-filled capsule – the contents of which are inhaled directly into the patient's lungs using a capsule-puncturing device equipped with a mouthpiece for inhalation. Examples include Advair® Diskus, Serevent® Diskus, and Spiriva® HandiHaler.

TRANSDERMAL DRUG DELIVERY SYSTEMS

Certain medications have special properties that enable them to cross the skin and enter the bloodstream. When these drugs are manufactured as skin patches, we call them transdermal drug delivery systems. Examples include Transderm Scop® for motion sickness, Ortho Evra® for birth control, Vivelle-Dot® for symptoms of menopause, Nitro-Dur® for angina, and Duragesic® for chronic pain. These dosage forms are known for their convenience. Most patches contain enough medication to last for several days.

SUPPOSITORIES AND INSERTS

Suppositories are solid under refrigeration and, in most cases, at room temperature, but melt at normal body temperature. There are different types of suppositories, but rectal suppositories are the most common. Rectal suppositories deliver medication directly to the rectum for one of two purposes. #1 To remain in the colon for treatment of a local condition, such as hemorrhoid pain or constipation, or #2 To be absorbed from the colon into the bloodstream for treatment of a systemic condition, such as a seizure or nausea and vomiting. An example of a rectal suppository for a local condition is the Tucks® suppository for hemorrhoids. For a systemic condition, an example is Phenadoz® suppositories for nausea and vomiting.

THERAPEUTIC EQUIVALENCE

Prescribers often issue prescriptions for brand name drug products, but we help patients save a lot of money by dispensing generic equivalents. Another term for "generic equivalent" is "therapeutic equivalent." Compared to a brand product, the generic or therapeutic equivalent is equal in terms of strength, quality, performance, safety, intended use, dosage form, route of administration, and rate and extent of absorption (pretty much every category that matters from a medical and scientific standpoint). The only difference between a brand product and a generic equivalent is the identity of the manufacturer and the composition of inactive ingredients (e.g., fillers, binders, and color additives).

THE FEDERAL ORANGE BOOK

Official Title: Approved Drug Products with Therapeutic Equivalence Evaluations

DETERMINATION OF THERAPEUTIC EQUIVALENCE

The Federal Orange Book contains a listing of "TE codes" (therapeutic equivalence codes) for generic drug products. Products with a TE code beginning with the letter A are deemed to be therapeutically equivalent to the brand name product. Pharmacists commonly refer to these products as "A-rated generics."

EXAMPLE SCENARIO

You receive a prescription for Lipitor® over the telephone. Should you dispense brand name Lipitor® or the generic equivalent, atorvastatin?

Atorvastatin. If the prescriber (or his/her agent) expressly stated that the brand name is necessary and substitution is not permitted, then it would have been appropriate to dispense the brand name version instead.

NARROW THERAPEUTIC INDEX DRUGS

Carbamazepine   Cyclosporine   Digoxin   Lithium   Phenytoin   Tacrolimus   Theophylline   Warfarin

There is no official federal list of narrow therapeutic index (NTI) drugs; however, a few common examples are listed above. NTI drugs require careful dose titration and patient monitoring for safe and effective use. For a drug to be considered to have a "narrow therapeutic index," one of the following two conditions must apply:
- There is less than a 2-fold difference between the median lethal dose (LD50) and the median effective dose (ED50).
- There is less than a 2-fold difference between the minimum toxic concentration (MTC) and the minimum effective concentration (MEC).

Note: ED50 is the dose that produces the desired effect in 50% of the population,
and LD50 is the dose that is lethal in 50% of the population.

TRUE OR FALSE

A BRAND NAME NARROW THERAPEUTIC INDEX DRUG SHOULD NOT BE SUBSTITUTED WITH A GENERIC DRUG.
It depends. The pharmacist must use professional judgment combined with regulatory knowledge to make the final determination in any generic substitution decision.

PROPER MEDICATION STORAGE

Most medications have specific storage requirements or manufacturer-recommended storage conditions that must be met to ensure the product remains stable and effective until the expiration date. Many environmental factors can negatively affect the chemical structure of the active ingredient(s) or disrupt the physical properties of the medium used to deliver the drug into the body (e.g., the drug delivery device or the inactive ingredients used to formulate the drug product). The most common examples of these deleterious environmental factors include temperature, humidity/ moisture, and sunlight.

- Temperature
    - Temperature can destroy the chemical and physical properties of a drug product. Study the chart below to learn how terms used in a manufacturer's product packaging like "keep cool" or "store at room temperature" can be translated into quantitative temperature ranges.

- Humidity/Moisture
    - Humidity and moisture can also destroy the chemical and physical properties of a drug product. Study the chart below to learn how terms used in product packaging like "store in a dry place" or "protect from moisture" can be translated into quantitative values.

- Sunlight
    - Sunlight is abundant in ultraviolet (UV) light, which has the capacity to change the chemical structure of the active and inactive ingredients that form the drug product. This is why pharmacies use amber vials/containers to dispense medication.

TEMPERATURE RANGES	
Frozen (Freezer)	-25°C to -10°C (-13°F to 14°F)
Cold (Refrigerator)	2°C to 8°C (36°F to 46°F)
Cool	8°C to 15°C (46°F to 59°F)
Room Temperature	20°C to 25°C (68°F to 77°F)
Warm	30°C to 40°C (86°F to 104°F)
Excessive Heat	> 40°C (> 104°F)

HUMIDITY RANGES	
Store in a Dry Place	Average Relative Humidity < or = 40%
Protect from Moisture	Relative Humidity < or = 60%*

*Defined by the World Health Organization (WHO) Technical Report Series.

DRUG PRODUCT	SPECIAL STORAGE REQUIREMENT
Nitrostat® (nitroglycerin sublingual tablets)	Do not remove tablets from the original container. Nitroglycerin is a volatile substance that quickly converts from solid to gas. When stored outside of the original container, the nitroglycerin will evaporate from the tablet. For this reason, it is important to keep nitroglycerin tablets tightly sealed in the original container (usually a small glass vial with a metal lid).
Pradaxa® (dabigatran oral capsules)	Pradaxa® is available in a bottle or blister packs. For the bottle, it is important not to remove the capsules from their original container until immediately prior to use. The drug is quickly destroyed by humidity in the air. The Pradaxa® bottle is equipped with a special cap that contains a desiccant (drying agent). Once the bottle is opened, the capsules inside expire after 4 months. For the blister packs, do not remove a capsule from the blister pack until immediately prior to use.
Xalatan® (latanoprost eye drops)	Refrigerate (2°–8°C) until opened. Once opened, latanoprost eye drops can be stored at room temperature (up to 25°C) for 6 weeks.
Insulin (all types and brands)	Refrigerate (2°–8°C) until first use. Once the rubber stopper of the vial is punctured, it can be stored either in the refrigerator or at room temperature for up to 28 days. After 28 days, sterility cannot be guaranteed.
Nitropress® (sodium nitroprusside injection)	Sodium nitroprusside is quickly deactivated upon exposure to light. To prevent light exposure, the medication comes in a small cardboard box containing a dark amber glass vial of sodium nitroprusside 50 mg/2 mL solution and an opaque light protective sleeve. The vial should only be removed from the box just prior to admixture. Once admixed, the IV infusion bag containing sodium nitroprusside must be placed in the opaque light protective sleeve to prevent exposure to light.

Consequences of Inappropriate Storage – Select Examples:

PRODUCT	CONSEQUENCE
Aerosols *Inhalers* - ProAir®, Ventolin®, Xopenex®, Qvar®, Symbicort® *Rectal Aerosols* - ProctoFoam®, ProctoFoam®-HC *Topical Aerosols* - Kenalog® spray, Tinactin® powder spray	Excessive heat can cause an aerosol container to burst/explode. When used at cool or colder temperatures, aerosol canisters tend to deliver less medication, resulting in sub-optimal drug delivery.
Insulin Levemir®, Lantus®, Humulin N®, Novolin N®, Humulin R®, Novolin R®, Humalog®, NovoLog®, Apidra® (and all other forms of insulin)	Insulin is a protein, which is a large molecule whose effectiveness is dependent upon its complex chemical structure. Proteins, such as insulin, have a rather delicate chemical structure. Temperature extremes (heat and cold) and physical shaking can destroy the chemical structure of proteins, rendering them inactive. Additionally, insulin is delivered in a sterile liquid medium as an injection. Warmth and excessive heat promote microbial contamination of the liquid medium, rendering the preparation unsafe for injection.
Suppositories Anucort-HC™ suppositories, Canasa® suppositories, Phenadoz™ suppositories, Glycerin suppositories	A suppository should be maintained in its individual wrapping until directly prior to insertion to protect the dosage form from humidity and moisture in the surrounding environment. If stored outside of their packaging, the suppositories can adhere to one another. Heat and moisture can cause the suppositories to melt and lose form.
Ointments Bactroban® Ointment, Mycolog®-II Ointment, Cortizone-10® Ointment	Warm environments and excessive heat can cause product separation.

Note: The bathroom is one of the worst places to store medication. Why? Hot baths and/or showers create steam (moisture and heat can destroy the ingredients).

INCOMPATIBILITIES RELATED TO NONSTERILE COMPOUNDING AND RECONSTITUTION

Water can accelerate the expiration of pharmaceutical products. To extend the shelf-life of certain products that would otherwise expire rapidly, some drugs are supplied as a dry powder for reconstitution. One common example is Amoxicillin for Oral Suspension.

"RECONSTITUTION" IS THE PROCESS OF RESTORING A DRIED PRODUCT TO ITS ORIGINAL LIQUID STATE THROUGH THE ADDITION OF WATER

When reconstituting any product, it is critical to keep in mind that the volume of diluent (typically sterile water) that must be added to the powder will vary based on the product and will always be lower than the final desired volume after reconstitution. For example, if the final volume of the reconstituted product should be 100 mL, then you should expect to add less than 100 mL of diluent during the reconstitution process. This is because the powdered drug occupies some volume. Another important point to remember is that every product contains detailed instructions for reconstitution directly on the package label. Follow these instructions carefully. If too much diluent is added to the powder, then the actual concentration of medication in the container will be lower than that displayed on the label, causing the patient to receive a lower-than-expected dose. Likewise, if too little diluent is added to the powder, then the actual concentration of medication in the container will be higher than that displayed on the label, causing the patient to receive a higher-than-expected dose. Both scenarios can lead to patient harm.

EXAMPLE

Amoxicillin for Oral Suspension 400 mg/5 mL (volume 50 mL when reconstituted) is supplied in a small plastic bottle containing amoxicillin powder for reconstitution. The instructions for reconstitution appearing on the label are as follows: "Tap bottle to loosen powder. Add approximately 1/3 of the total volume of water to reconstitute the powder (**total = 34 mL**). Sake vigorously. Add remaining water. Shake vigorously again."

CHECK FOR INCOMPATIBILITIES

When reconstituting or compounding any product, it is important to keep an eye out for signs of physical or chemical incompatibility, such as:

- Precipitate formation (solid particles)
- Gas formation (bubbles)
- Turbidity (cloudiness)
- Color changes

BEYOND-USE DATE AND AUXILIARY LABELS

Once the product has been reconstituted, be sure to write the beyond-use date on the container. This information also appears directly on the package label. For instance, in our amoxicillin example, the label states, "Discard unused portion after 14 days." Also, affix auxiliary labels, such as "Keep Refrigerated" and "Shake Well" (if necessary). Suspensions must be shaken prior to administration, but solutions need not be shaken. See the next page for more information regarding auxiliary labels.

AUXILIARY LABELS

In many cases, a prescriber's directions for use fall short of providing all of the details necessary for proper use and storage of the prescribed medication. This is where auxiliary labels come in. By affixing the relevant auxiliary labels, pharmacists and pharmacy technicians can help fill in the information gap. The pharmacy computers may be programmed to print the relevant auxiliary labels with each prescription label; however, sometimes they may need to be added manually. See the illustration below for an example of a retail prescription label with three auxiliary labels (located to the right of the barcode).

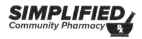

SIMPLIFIED ℞
Community Pharmacy

4321 Easy St. New York, NY 10001
Telephone: 555-0198

Rx# 0012875   B. Smith, MD   Filled   09/30/2021
John Doe
321 Old Dirt Rd, New York, NY 10001

TAKE ONE TABLET BY MOUTH TWICE DAILY WITH A MEAL

METOPROLOL 50 MG TABLETS   **QTY: 60**
Manufactured by SIMPLIFIED PHARMA

Expires 03/31/2023

2 Refills   RPh: DH

| TAKE WITH FOOD |
| MAY CAUSE DIZZINESS |
| DO NOT DRINK ALCOHOLIC BEVERAGES WHILE TAKING THIS MEDICATION |

Caution: Federal law prohibits the transfer of this drug to any person other than the patient for whom it was prescribed

KNOWLEDGE AREA #2
FEDERAL REQUIREMENTS

WHEN FEDERAL LAW AND STATE LAW DIFFER, THE MORE RESTRICTIVE LAW APPLIES

For example, federal law typically requires pharmacies to maintain prescription records for at least two (2) years; meanwhile, many states require a longer prescription record maintenance period. In such cases, a pharmacy must comply with whichever prescription record maintenance requirement is longer.

ROLE OF GOVERNMENT AGENCIES

State Board of Pharmacy
Each state has a separate board of pharmacy that is responsible for protecting the health, safety, and welfare of its citizens in matters related to the practice of pharmacy, which is accomplished through the enforcement of pharmacy laws and regulations. State boards of pharmacy are also in charge of regulating traditional compounding pharmacies.

Food and Drug Administration (FDA)
The FDA enforces drug manufacturing laws and regulates prescription drug advertising, which is known as "direct to consumer" (DTC) advertising. The FDA also regulates large-scale compounding facilities.

Drug Enforcement Administration (DEA)
The DEA enforces the federal Controlled Substances Act (CSA) and makes decisions regarding the classification of certain drugs as controlled substances.

Occupational Safety and Health Administration (OSHA)
OSHA enforces occupational health and safety laws. They play a major role in reducing the risk of employee exposure to bloodborne pathogens. This is particularly relevant for places where employees routinely work with needles, as is the case in pharmacies that perform sterile compounding or offer immunizations and vaccinations.

Federal Trade Commission (FTC)
The FTC regulates advertising for over-the-counter drugs, medical devices, cosmetics, and food products.

Note: The government classifies vitamins and herbal supplements as food products.

HANDLING AND DISPOSAL OF HAZARDOUS DRUGS

A hazardous drug is a medication that can cause harm to human or animal life. For example, exposure to a hazardous drug may cause reproductive toxicity, organ damage, birth defects, and/or cancer. Cancer chemotherapy agents, antiviral agents, immunosuppressants, hormones, and certain anticonvulsants make up the majority of drugs that are classified as "hazardous."

A hazardous drug becomes "hazardous waste" when it expires, is spilled, is present as a residue, or is otherwise no longer needed. There are four categories of hazardous waste:
- F list (non-specific source)
- K list (source-specific)
- P list (acutely hazardous discarded commercial chemicals)
- U list (toxic discarded commercial chemicals)

Hazardous pharmaceutical wastes appear on the P and U lists. Drugs appearing on the "P list" (e.g., warfarin, epinephrine, phentermine, nitroglycerin) are acutely hazardous; whereas, drugs appearing on the "U list" (e.g., various cancer chemotherapy agents) are toxic.

WHY DO HAZARDOUS DRUGS EXIST?

Consider a patient with cancer. Cancer, if left untreated, could grow and spread very quickly. Now imagine that there is a drug that could slow and potentially stop the cancer growth, but this drug is known to be toxic to the liver. For the patient with cancer, the benefit of treating cancer is likely to outweigh the risk of liver toxicity.

When handling hazardous drugs, healthcare workers should follow _____ and any recommendations included in the manufacturer's _____.
- Standard precautions
- Safety data sheet (SDS)

What standard precautions must be followed by healthcare workers when handling hazardous drugs?
- Store hazardous drugs in a well-ventilated area separate from all other inventory.
- Wear chemotherapy gloves whenever handling hazardous drugs (e.g., when receiving, stocking, counting, preparing for administration, and disposing of).
- Perform sterile compounding activities with hazardous drugs in an ISO class 5 biological safety cabinet or compounding aseptic containment isolator.
  Note: The safety cabinet or containment isolator used for compounding hazardous drugs must be physically separate from other sterile compounding preparation areas.
- Wear appropriate personal protective equipment (PPE) when compounding products that contain hazardous drugs.
  - Gown.
  - Face mask.
  - Eye protection. *
  - Hair cover.
  - Shoe covers.
  - Double-gloving with sterile chemotherapy gloves. *

  *Precautions not routinely recommended for compounding non-hazardous sterile drug products.

Why must healthcare workers follow standard precautions when handling hazardous drugs?
To avoid exposing to healthy individuals to the risks associated with a drug from which they will derive no therapeutic benefit.

What organizations provide information regarding the storage, handling, and disposal of hazardous drugs?
- United States Pharmacopoeia (USP)
- American Society of Health-System Pharmacists (ASHP)
- National Institute for Occupational Safety and Health (NIOSH)
- Occupational Safety and Health Administration (OSHA)

What information is provided in a product's safety data sheet (SDS)?
- Chemical and physical properties.
- Health, safety, fire, and environmental hazards.
- Information on what to do if the product is accidentally spilled.

Safety Data Sheets are for _____ & _____.
- Workers that will potentially be exposed to chemicals.
- Emergency response personnel (e.g., firefighters).

Who is responsible for making SDSs available to employees?
The employer.

What type of container must be used for disposal of needles and syringes with hazardous drug residue?
Chemotherapy sharps container.

How does one distinguish a standard sharps container from a chemotherapy sharps container?
Standard sharps containers are red; whereas, chemotherapy sharps containers are yellow.

What is the purpose of a black pharmaceutical waste container?
Black pharmaceutical waste containers are used for the disposal of bulk hazardous drug waste (e.g., disposal of a half-empty vial of a cancer chemotherapy drug).

All areas where hazardous drugs are routinely handled must contain:
- Hazardous drug spill kits
- Containment bags
- Disposal containers

REVIEW OF PHARMACEUTICAL WASTE CONTAINERS

	Red Container	Yellow Container	Black Container
Standard Sharps Waste	✓		
Sharps Waste with Hazardous Drug Residue		✓	
Bulk Hazardous Drug Waste			✓

What supplies appear in a hazardous drug spill kit?

- Material to absorb about 1,000 mL of liquid
  - Plastic-backed, absorbent spill cleanup pads
  - Disposable towels
- Personal protective equipment (PPE)
  - Two (2) pairs of gloves
  - Gown
  - Shoe covers
  - Face shield
- Two (2) or more sealable plastic hazardous waste disposal bags
- One (1) disposable scooper and one (1) puncture-resistant container for collecting and disposing of broken glass.

Note: all spill cleanup materials must be disposed of as hazardous waste.

What steps should be taken in the event of exposure to a hazardous drug by direct skin or eye contact?

- Call for help (if necessary).
- Remove any contaminated clothing.
- Wash the affected eye(s) with water for at least 15 minutes.
- Clean the affected skin with soap and water. Rinse well.
- Seek medical attention and document the exposure.

HAZARDOUS DRUGS – SELECT EXAMPLES

DRUG CLASS	GENERIC DRUG NAME
Cancer Chemotherapy	Anastrozole
	Bicalutamide
	Cisplatin
	Exemestane
	5-Fluorouracil
	Letrozole
	Mercaptopurine
	Methotrexate
	Oxaliplatin
	Tamoxifen
	Vinblastine
	Vincristine
Antiviral Agents	Abacavir
	Entecavir
	Ganciclovir
	Valganciclovir
	Zidovudine
Immune System Suppressants	Azathioprine
	Cyclosporine
	Mycophenolate
	Sirolimus
	Tacrolimus

Source: Connor TH, Burroughs GE, McDiarmid MA, Mead KR, Power LA, Reed LD. NIOSH Alert: preventing occupational exposures to antineoplastic and other hazardous drugs in health care settings. Atlanta. DHHS (NIOSH) Publication. 2004:1-50.

POISON PREVENTION PACKAGING ACT OF 1970 (PPPA)

✓ Enacted to reduce the incidence of death and serious injury caused when children access and consume medications and other dangerous household substances (e.g., household cleaning agents).

✓ Requires most medications to be dispensed in child-resistant packages (e.g., child safety caps on prescriptions dispensed from a pharmacy).

✓ Containers must be **significantly difficult** for children under 5-years-old to open, but not difficult for adults.

✓ Exceptions to the child-resistant packaging requirement include:
  - o Nitroglycerin Sublingual Tablets
  - o Steroid Dose Packs
  - o Aerosols
  - o Birth Control Pills
  - o Female Hormone Replacement Drugs

NITROGLYCERIN SUBLINGUAL TABLETS ARE THE MOST NOTEWORTHY EXCEPTION TO THE CHILD-RESISTANT PACKAGING REQUIREMENT.

If an adult has difficulty with or is unable to open a prescription bottle equipped with a child safety cap (e.g., due to arthritis), then the patient may request an easy-open cap (also referred to as a "snap cap"). The prescribing practitioner may also request an easy-open cap on behalf of the patient by making a notation on the face of the prescription.

OMNIBUS BUDGET RECONCILIATION ACT OF 1990 (OBRA '90)

✓ Requires pharmacists to perform prospective drug utilization reviews (DURs) and offer to counsel Medicaid patients. When performing a DUR, the pharmacist should look for things like...
  - o Therapeutic duplications.
  - o Drug-disease contraindications.
  - o Drug-drug interactions.
  - o Incorrect doses.
  - o Inappropriate duration of treatment.
  - o Drug-allergy interactions.
  - o Clinical abuse/misuse.

✓ To contract with Medicaid, pharmacies must implement standards to provide counseling to Medicaid patients. The "offer to counsel" requirement does not apply in inpatient settings.

✓ Pharmacists must make a reasonable effort to keep patient profiles up to date.

✓ This specific law pertains only to Medicaid patients, but states have expanded it to apply to all patients.

HEALTH INSURANCE PORTABILITY & ACCOUNTABILITY ACT (HIPAA)

HIPAA is legislation that protects the privacy and security of patient medical records and health information ("protected health information" or "PHI").

HIPAA PRIVACY RULE
- ✓ Limits the use and disclosure of protected health information (PHI) to the "minimum necessary."
- ✓ Provides an option for the patient to obtain a copy of their health record and request corrections.

HIPAA SECURITY RULE
- ✓ Requires various administrative, physical, and technical safeguards to ensure the confidentiality, integrity, and overall security of protected health information, including electronic medical records.
- ✓ Outlines national standards for healthcare providers, insurance companies, and healthcare financial claim processing companies to protect the privacy of individual health information.

HIPAA BREACH NOTIFICATION RULE
- ✓ If protected health information has been exposed to unauthorized individuals, the affected patient(s) must be notified.

WHEN "MINIMUM NECESSARY USE AND DISCLOSURE" DOES NOT APPLY
- Disclosures to a healthcare provider for treatment
- Disclosures to the patient upon request
- Disclosures authorized by the patient
- Disclosures necessary to comply with other laws
- Disclosures to the Department of Health and Human Services (HHS) for a compliance investigation, review, or enforcement

PRACTICAL MEASURES FOR PROTECTING PATIENT HEALTH INFORMATION
- Maintain a reasonable distance between the patient with whom you are speaking and other people in the area to prevent sensitive information from being overheard.
- Speak loudly enough for the patient to hear you, but not loud enough for bystanders to hear.
- Do not shout to a patient when discussing PHI, such as medication names, medical conditions, date of birth, address, and other sensitive information.
- Never gossip about a patient and their medical information.
- Do not disclose PHI to anyone over the phone who is not legally authorized to access the information.

FEDERAL FOOD, DRUG & COSMETIC ACT (FD&C ACT)

The first federal law to regulate drug products was the Pure Food and Drug Act of 1906. This legislation addressed purity but did not address safety or prohibit false claims. In 1938, the Pure Food and Drug Act was replaced by the Food, Drug, and Cosmetic Act (FD&C Act). This new legislation required drug manufacturers to provide the FDA with evidence of safety by submitting a New Drug Application (NDA); however, if action was not taken by the FDA within 60 days, the drug was automatically approved. The FD&C Act has undergone several amendments since it was first passed in 1938. In this section of the study guide, we highlight key amendments and their impact on the practice of pharmacy.

DURHAM-HUMPHREY AMENDMENT (1951)
✓ Drug products are separated into two categories: over the counter and prescription-only ("legend drugs").
✓ Legend drug labels must state, "Caution: Federal law prohibits dispensing without a prescription."

KEFAUVER HARRIS AMENDMENT (1962)
✓ Passed in reaction to "The Thalidomide Tragedy," which took place between 1957 – 1961.
✓ To obtain FDA approval for a drug, manufacturers must provide substantial evidence of safety and efficacy.
✓ Previously, New Drug Applications gained automatic approval after 60 days if the FDA did not take action. With this amendment, manufacturers must prove safety regardless of the time frame.
✓ In the past, manufacturers were not required to prove efficacy.

FEDERAL ANTI-TAMPERING ACT (1982)
✓ Passed in reaction to the "Chicago Tylenol® Murders," which took place in 1982.
✓ Over the counter (OTC) drug products must have a tamper-evident seal.

PRESCRIPTION DRUG MARKETING ACT OF 1987 (PDMA)
✓ Banned the selling/purchasing/trading of prescription drug samples.

DIETARY SUPPLEMENT HEALTH AND EDUCATION ACT OF 1994 (DSHEA)
✓ Dietary supplements (e.g., vitamins, minerals, herbal supplements) are classified as "food" since they supplement the diet. As a result, manufacturers can market dietary supplements without FDA review.
✓ For drug products, a manufacturer must prove safety before entering the market, but for food products, the FDA must prove a lack of safety to be able to take a product off the market.

FOOD AND DRUG ADMINISTRATION MODERNIZATION ACT OF 1997 (FDAMA)
✓ The statement required to appear on legend drug labels per the Durham-Humphrey Amendment ("Caution: Federal law prohibits dispensing without a prescription") could be shortened to "Rx only."

CONTROLLED SUBSTANCE SCHEDULES

SCHEDULE I CONTROLLED SUBSTANCES
Examples: GHB, heroin

- No accepted medical use
- Not legal for prescribing purposes
- High potential for abuse
- Unsafe

SCHEDULE II CONTROLLED SUBSTANCES
Examples: MS Contin® (morphine sulfate ER), Roxicodone® (oxycodone)

- Accepted medical use
- Available by prescription only
- High potential for abuse
- High potential for physical/psychological dependence

SCHEDULE III CONTROLLED SUBSTANCES
Examples: AndroGel® (testosterone), Marinol® (dronabinol), Subutex® (buprenorphine)

- Accepted medical use
- Available by prescription only
- Moderate potential for abuse
- Moderate-low potential for physical/psychological dependence

SCHEDULE IV CONTROLLED SUBSTANCES
Examples: Valium® (diazepam), Xanax® (alprazolam), Provigil® (modafinil)

- Accepted medical use
- Available by prescription only
- Mild potential for abuse
- Mild potential for physical/psychological dependence

SCHEDULE V CONTROLLED SUBSTANCES
Examples: Lomotil® (diphenoxylate/atropine), Cheratussin® AC (guaifenesin/codeine)

- Accepted medical use
- Available by prescription; limited quantities of certain C-V drugs known as **"exempt narcotics"** are available without a prescription in some states
- Low potential for abuse
- Low potential for physical/psychological dependence

COMMON CONTROLLED SUBSTANCES CATEGORIZED BY SCHEDULE

It is important to recognize the schedule to which a controlled substance belongs, as regulations vary based on the schedule. See below for a list of the most recognized and prescribed controlled substances categorized by schedule. Note that the information below was derived from the federal Controlled Substances Act (CSA). The laws in your state result in more stringent scheduling of certain substances; however, questions on the PTCB® exam pertain to federal law only. Generic names are listed with brand names in parenthesis (when available).

SCHEDULE I (C-I) CONTROLLED SUBSTANCES

- gamma-hydroxybutyric acid (GHB)
- heroin
- lysergic acid diethylamide (LSD)
- marijuana
- 3,4-methylenedioxymethamphetamine (MDMA)

SCHEDULE II (C-II) CONTROLLED SUBSTANCES

C-II Opioids:
- codeine
- hydrocodone (including combination products)
- morphine (MS Contin®, Roxanol®)
- meperidine (Demerol®)
- methadone (Dolophine®, Methadose®)
- fentanyl (Duragesic®)
- hydromorphone (Dilaudid®, Exalgo®)
- oxycodone (Roxicodone®, Oxycontin®)
- oxymorphone (Numorphan®, Opana®)

C-II Stimulants:
- amphetamine/dextroamphetamine (Adderall®)
- cocaine
- methamphetamine (Desoxyn®)
- methylphenidate (Concerta®, Metadate®, Methylin®, Ritalin®)

C-II Depressants:
- amobarbital (Amytal®)
- pentobarbital (Nembutal®)
- secobarbital (Seconal®)

C-II Hallucinogens:
- nabilone (Cesamet®)

SCHEDULE III (C-III) CONTROLLED SUBSTANCES

C-III Opioids:
- buprenorphine (Buprenex®, Subutex®)
- buprenorphine/naloxone (Suboxone®)
- camphorated tincture of opium (Paregoric®)
- codeine* (e.g., Tylenol® with codeine, Fioricet® with codeine)

*Categorized as a C-III controlled when used in limited quantities in combination with other medications.

C-III Mixed Opioid Agonist/Antagonists:
- nalorphine (Nalline®)

C-III Stimulants:
- benzphetamine (Didrex®, Regimex)
- phendimetrazine (Bontril®)

C-III Depressants:
- barbituric acid and its derivatives
- ketamine (Ketalar®)

The following Schedule II depressants are considered Schedule III when they exist in a compound, mixture, or suppository form:
- amobarbital
- pentobarbital
- secobarbital

C-III Anabolic Steroids:
All anabolic steroids are C-III according to federal law.
- testosterone (AndroGel®, Testim®, Axiron®, Depo-Testosterone®)
- oxandrolone (Oxandrin®)

C-III Hallucinogens:
- dronabinol (Marinol®)

SCHEDULE IV (C-IV) CONTROLLED SUBSTANCES

C-IV Depressants (Benzodiazepines):
- alprazolam (Xanax®)
- chlordiazepoxide (Librium®)
- clonazepam (Klonopin®)
- clorazepate (Tranxene®)
- diazepam (Valium®, Diastat®)
- estazolam (Prosom®)
- flurazepam (Dalmane®)
- lorazepam (Ativan®)
- midazolam (Versed®)
- temazepam (Restoril®)

C-IV Depressants (Non-Benzodiazepines):
- eszopiclone (Lunesta®)
- zaleplon (Sonata®)
- zolpidem (Ambien®)
- phenobarbital (Luminal®)
- carisoprodol (Soma®)
- tramadol (Ultram®)

C-IV Mixed Opioid Agonist/Antagonists:
- butorphanol (Stadol®)
- pentazocine (Talwin®)

C-IV Stimulants:
- modafinil (Provigil®)
- phentermine (Adipex-P®, Suprenza™)
- phentermine/topiramate (Qsymia®)
- sibutramine (Meridia®)

SCHEDULE V (C-V) CONTROLLED SUBSTANCES

C-V Opioids:
- codeine preparations (≤200 mg/100 mL or 100 g; Robitussin® AC)
- diphenoxylate with atropine (≤2.5 mg/25 mcg atropine; Lomotil®)
- opium preparations (≤100 mg/100 mL or 100 g)

C-V Depressants:
- pregabalin (Lyrica®)
- lacosamide (Vimpat®)
- brivaracetam (Briviact®)
- cannabidiol drugs with ≤0.1% (w/w) residual tetrahydrocannabinol

---

For a comprehensive list of controlled substances, please visit
<http://www.deadiversion.usdoj.gov/schedules/orangebook/e_cs_sched.pdf>

FEDERAL CONTROLLED SUBSTANCES ACT

The federal Controlled Substances Act (CSA) is located in Title 21 of the Code of Federal Regulations, Part 1300 through 1321 (21 CFR § 1300 – 1321). This section of the study guide highlights and summarizes key points from the CSA. Citations are provided in parenthesis.

✓ The goal of the CSA is to prevent illicit drug use and distribution while allowing for legitimate medical use.

✓ This law is also known as the "Comprehensive Drug Abuse Prevention and Control Act."

✓ The Drug Enforcement Administration (DEA) is responsible for enforcing the CSA.

Note: When reading the original text of the controlled substances act, it is important to recognize that the term "practitioner" is used to describe physicians, dentists, veterinarians, scientific investigators, **pharmacies**, hospitals, or anyone else permitted to handle controlled substances. (21 CFR § 802)

ACCEPTABLE CONTROLLED SUBSTANCE PRESCRIPTION FORMATS
(21 CFR § 1306.11 & 1306.21)

C-II: Written or Electronic. *
C-III – IV: Written, Verbal, Faxed, or Electronic.
C-V: Written, Verbal, Faxed, Electronic, or OTC. **

* Special cases for Schedule II prescriptions:
   #1 EMERGENCY C-II PRESCRIPTIONS – VERBAL PRESCRIPTION ORDERS PERMITTED
   - Schedule II prescription may be dispensed pursuant to verbal order only in an emergency
   - Prescription must be communicated directly from the prescriber to the pharmacist
   - Pharmacist must immediately reduce the verbal prescription to writing
   - If prescriber is unknown, pharmacist must make a reasonable effort to verify validity.
   - Quantity must be limited to the amount adequate to treat the patient during the emergency period
      o The law does not provide specific quantity limits
   - Prescriber must deliver a written hardcopy prescription to the dispensing pharmacy within 7 days
   - The hardcopy prescription should be attached to and kept on file with the verbal order
   #2 FAXED C-II PRESCRIPTIONS
   - Faxed prescription may serve as the "original prescription" for these three (3) patient populations:
      1) Hospice patients
      2) Home infusion patients
      3) Long-term care facility residents
   - For all other patient populations, faxed C-II prescriptions may be filled, but cannot be dispensed until the patient presents the original prescription. The pharmacist must verify the original prescription against the faxed prescription prior to dispensing. The pharmacy must keep the original prescription for recordkeeping purposes.

** Limited quantities of a controlled substance may be dispensed without a prescription if state law permits.

ELECTRONIC CONTROLLED SUBSTANCE PRESCRIPTIONS (21 CFR § 1306.08)

Federal law permits e-prescribing of C-II through C-V controlled substances as long as the prescriber and pharmacy use e-prescription software that meets DEA requirements.

CONTROLLED SUBSTANCE PRESCRIPTION REFILLS

C-II: Refills are **not** permitted (21 CFR § 1306.12)
C-III – IV: Up to 5 refills (21 CFR § 1306.22)
C-V: No maximum

CONTROLLED SUBSTANCE PRESCRIPTION EXPIRATION
C-II: No expiration
C-III – IV: Expires 6 months after the date written (21 CFR § 1306.22)
C-V: No expiration

CONTROLLED SUBSTANCE PRESCRIPTION PARTIAL FILLS
C-II: Permitted at the request of the patient or prescriber as long as the remainder is filled within 30 days. If the partial fill is for an oral emergency prescription, then the remainder must be filled within 72 hours. If the remainder is not filled within the respective time frames described above, then the remainder is void, and the prescriber must be notified. * (21 CFR § 1306.13 & S. 524 (CARA of 2016))
C-III – V: Permitted with no time limit for completion; however, keep in mind that C-III and C-IV prescriptions expire 6 months after the date written.
* For long-term care or terminally ill patients, multiple partial fills for Schedule II prescriptions are Are permitted for up to 60 days from the date written. (21 CFR § 1306.13)

THE 5 REFILL LIMIT FOR C-III AND C-IV PRESCRIPTIONS
Mary has a prescription for 30 tablets of Ativan® with instructions to take 1 tablet by mouth nightly as needed with 5 refills. Imagine that Mary requests just 15 tablets each time she has the prescription filled.

In scenarios like the one described above, a pharmacist may consider the following:
Schedule III & IV controlled substance prescriptions are limited to 5 refills within 6 months from the date issued. If Mary receives 15 tablets per fill, must she forfeit the prescribed quantity that remains after the 5th fill?

The answer is *no*. In this case, the first 15 tablets are considered to be a "partial fill." The next 15 tablets would represent a completion of the partial fill. This cycle would continue until the patients receives all 180 tablets prescribed, or until the prescription expires, whichever comes first.

MAIN POINT: The number of times a C-III or C-IV prescription is filled is not important. What is important?

#1 the prescriber cannot authorize more than 5 refills.
#2 the patient cannot receive a quantity above that which is prescribed.

TRANSFERRING CONTROLLED SUBSTANCE PRESCRIPTION ORDERS FOR REFILL
C-II: Transfers are **not** permitted.
C-III – V: May be transferred to another pharmacy on a *one-time* basis between two licensed pharmacists. Transfers are unlimited for pharmacies that share a real-time, online database. (21 CFR § 1306.25)

MAINTENANCE OF CONTROLLED SUBSTANCE PRESCRIPTION RECORDS
C-II: Must be stored separately from all other prescription records. (21 CFR § 1304.04)
C-III – V: Must be stored either separate from all other prescription records or marked in the lower right corner with the letter "C" at least 1-inch high in red ink and stored in the same file with non-controlled substance prescription records. (21 CFR § 1304.04)

CONTROLLED SUBSTANCE STORAGE & SECURITY
Controlled substances must be stored in a locked cabinet or dispersed among non-controlled stock in such a manner as to deter theft or diversion. (21 CFR § 1301.75)

DISTRIBUTING OR RECEIVING CONTROLLED SUBSTANCE INVENTORY
C-II: Use a **DEA Form 222** to document the transaction. * (21 CFR § 1305.03)
C-III – V: Use an **invoice** to document the transaction.
* The Controlled Substance Ordering System (CSOS) is an electronic alternative to the DEA Form 222.

THE "5% RULE" FOR PHARMACIES

Pharmacies that are registered with the DEA may distribute a limited number of controlled substance dosage units to another DEA-registered pharmacy or practitioner **without registering as a distributor**. The limit is 5% of the total number of controlled substance dosage units dispensed during one (1) calendar year.

TO DISPENSE A QUANTITY OF CONTROLLED SUBSTANCE DOSAGE UNITS IN EXCESS OF 5% OF THE TOTAL QUANTITY DISPENSED DURING ONE (1) CALENDAR YEAR, A PHARMACY MUST REGISTER AS A DISTRIBUTOR.

Records of distribution and receipt must be maintained for at least two (2) years.
- ✓ Executed DEA Form 222 for C-II drugs
- ✓ Invoices for C-III, IV, and V drugs

DISPOSAL OF CONTROLLED SUBSTANCE INVENTORY (21 CFR 1317.05)

Controlled substance inventory that is expired or otherwise unusable should be disposed of promptly by any of these methods:
- ✓ Destroy the substance on-site (i.e., in the pharmacy/facility) in the presence of a DEA agent or other authorized person.
    - o Permission from DEA must be obtained in advance. *
    - o Two (2) employees of the DEA registrant must witness the destruction. (21 CFR 1317.95)
    - o No specific method of destruction is required, but the drug must be rendered "non-retrievable."
    - o Document destruction on a DEA Form 41.
- ✓ Deliver the substance to a reverse distributor.
    - o Document the transaction on a DEA Form 222.
- ✓ For returns or recalls, deliver the substance to the source from which it was obtained.
    - o Document the transaction on a DEA Form 222.
- ✓ Request assistance from the Special Agent in Charge at the local DEA office.
    - o Submit DEA Form 41 to the Special Agent in Charge.
    - o Wait to receive disposal instructions.

* Practitioners (i.e., prescribers, pharmacies, and hospitals) that routinely dispose of controlled substances can obtain special authorization from the DEA to dispose of controlled substances without first obtaining permission. These practitioners must maintain disposal records and report a summary of disposal activities periodically to the DEA Special Agent in Charge.

CONTROLLED SUBSTANCE DRUG WASTAGE

According to a DEA letter to registrants that was written on September 9, 2014, destruction of controlled substance drug wastage in an institutional setting, such as that which is produced when a nurse administers only a fraction of a controlled substance from a pre-filled syringe, should be recorded in compliance with 21 CFR 1304.22(c). The destruction of controlled substance drug wastage in an institutional setting should **not** be recorded on a DEA Form 41.

DRUG TAKE-BACK EVENTS

Law enforcement, or anyone partnering with law enforcement, has the authority to conduct drug take-back events in which legally obtained Schedule II, III, IV, and V controlled substances (+/- other prescription drugs) are collected from patients to be properly destroyed. [21 CFR 1317.65]

OTHER KEY POINTS REGARDING CONTROLLED SUBSTANCES

- A controlled substance prescription must be issued for a legitimate medical purpose in the practitioner's usual course of professional practice. (21 CFR § 1306.04)
- The dispensing pharmacist shares a corresponding responsibility with the prescriber for proper prescribing and dispensing of controlled substances. (21 CFR § 1306.04)
- Post-dating prescriptions (i.e., writing an issue date on the prescription that is later than the actual date issued) is prohibited.
- Prescribers are allowed to issue multiple C-II prescriptions to the same patient for the same medication, as long as they indicate the earliest fill date on each prescription AND the total amount prescribed does not exceed a 90-day supply. (21 CFR § 1306.12)
- It is illegal for a patient to mail/ship controlled substances out of the country.
- Federal law places no limit on the number of dosage units of a controlled substance that can be authorized by prescription at one time.
- Verbal orders/prescriptions for controlled substances must be communicated directly **from the prescriber to the pharmacist.** To be clear, pharmacy technicians **cannot** accept oral prescriptions for controlled substances, and agents of the prescriber (e.g., nurses, medical assistants, and secretaries) **cannot** provide telephone authorization for controlled substance prescriptions. (21 CFR 1306.21)
- An agent of the prescriber (e.g., a nurse, medical assistant, or secretary) CAN fax a controlled substance prescription to the pharmacy as long as the prescription is manually signed by the prescriber before faxing. (21 CFR 1306.21)

REQUIRED INFORMATION FOR CONTROLLED SUBSTANCE PRESCRIPTION ORDERS
(21 CFR § 1306.05)

- ✓ Patient's Full Name & Address.
- ✓ Prescriber's Full Name & Address.
- ✓ Prescriber's DEA Number.
- ✓ Drug Name, Strength, & Dosage Form.
- ✓ Quantity Prescribed.
- ✓ Directions for Use.
- ✓ Date Issued.
- ✓ Prescriber's Signature (**not** required for verbal prescriptions).

DEA REGISTRATION

- ✓ Required for all practitioners who prescribe controlled substances and all entities involved in the production or distribution of controlled substances. Registrants receive a DEA number.
  - ✓ DEA registrations must be renewed once every 3 years.

OVER-THE-COUNTER CONTROLLED SUBSTANCE SALES (21 CFR § 1306.26)

Limited quantities of controlled substances may be dispensed without a prescription if state law permits.

LIMITS*

- ✓ 8 ounces (240 mL) of an opium-containing liquid drug product
- ✓ 4 ounces (120 mL) of a liquid that contains a controlled substance other than opium
- ✓ 48 dosage units of an opium-containing solid drug product
- ✓ 24 dosage units of a solid drug product that contains a controlled substance other than opium

*Limits per individual in any 48-hour period

RECORDKEEPING REQUIREMENTS

- ✓ Purchaser must be at least 18 years old
- ✓ Purchaser must furnish ID
- ✓ The pharmacy must record:
  - ○ Name & address of purchaser
  - ○ Name & quantity of controlled substance sold over the counter
  - ○ Date of sale
  - ○ Name or initials of dispensing pharmacist

Per 21 CFR § 1304.04, controlled substance records must be kept for at least 2 years

CONTROLLED SUBSTANCE INVENTORY REQUIREMENTS (21 CFR § 1304.11)

INITIAL INVENTORY
An initial inventory must be taken when a pharmacy first opens for business.

BIENNIAL INVENTORY
Entire controlled substance inventory must be counted at least once every 2 years.

NEWLY SCHEDULED DRUG OR CHANGE IN SCHEDULE OF A DRUG
When a drug is newly categorized as a controlled substance (or if the schedule of an existing controlled substance changes), the affected drug must be inventoried the day that the change takes effect.

INVENTORY COUNTING PROCEDURES

For C-II controlled substances, an **exact count** or measure of every container is required regardless of size.
For C-III, C-IV, and C-V controlled substances...
- ✓ An **estimate** or exact count is acceptable for open containers that hold ≤ 1,000 tablets or capsules.
- ✓ An **exact count** is required for open containers that hold >1,000 tablets or capsules.

NOTE: Controlled substance **drug samples** are not exempt from inventory requirements.
Per 21 CFR § 1304.04, controlled substance records must be kept for at least 2 years.

DEA FORMS

The Drug Enforcement Administration (DEA) is responsible for enforcing the federal Controlled Substances Act (CSA). The DEA's goal is to ensure that controlled substances are available for legitimate medical and research purposes while preventing illicit use and illegal distribution. To accomplish this, the DEA strictly monitors the manufacturing, distribution, and dispensing of controlled substances. Consequently, extensive documentation is required for the legitimate handling of controlled substances. To standardize recordkeeping procedures, the DEA provides preformatted forms for pharmacies and other individuals/entities that handle controlled substances. Use the chart below to memorize the titles of the most commonly used forms ("DEA Form Number") and their associated purposes.

FORM NUMBER	PURPOSE
DEA Form 41	For reporting the destruction of controlled substances.
DEA Form 104	For reporting a pharmacy closure or surrender of a pharmacy permit.
DEA Form 106	For reporting the loss or theft of controlled substances.
DEA Form 222	For ordering Schedule I & II controlled substances.
DEA Form 222a	For ordering an additional supply of DEA 222 forms.
DEA Form 224	For applying for a DEA registration number.
DEA Form 224a	For renewing DEA registration (renewal is required every 3 years).

In pharmacy, the most commonly used DEA form is the DEA Form 222. For that reason, pharmacists should be very familiar with this particular form and its use. See below for an outline of important details:
Each DEA Form 222 includes 2 carbon copies (the original, plus 2 attached copies):
1) The first page (the original) is brown.
   o Must be retained by the drug supplier.
2) The second page (the first carbon copy) is green.
   o Must be forwarded to the DEA by the drug supplier.
3) The third page (the second carbon copy) is blue.
   o Must be retained by the pharmacy.

MISTAKES CANNOT BE CORRECTED

In the event of an error, all copies of the DEA Form 222 must be voided and retained by the pharmacy.

EXAMPLE SCENARIO

When ordering Schedule II controlled substances for your pharmacy, what must you do with the first two pages (brown and green) of the DEA Form 222?

Give them to the supplier without separating them. For the form to be valid from the supplier's perspective, the brown and green copies must be intact with the carbon paper between them. The pharmacy must retain the third page (blue copy) of the form for recordkeeping purposes.

Note: Pharmacies must keep all controlled substance records (including executed DEA forms) for at least 2 years.

ELECTRONIC ALTERNATIVE TO THE DEA FORM 222

The Controlled Substance Ordering System (CSOS) is an electronic alternative to the DEA Form 222.

SUMMARY OF FEDERAL CONTROLLED SUBSTANCES ACT REQUIREMENTS

	SCHEDULE II	SCHEDULE III & IV	SCHEDULE V
DEA Registration	Required	Required	Required
Receiving Records	DEA Form 222	Invoices	Invoices
Accepted Prescription Formats	Written or Electronic	Written, Verbal, Faxed, or Electronic	Written, Verbal, Faxed, Electronic or OTC*
Refills	No	No more than 5 within 6 months	As authorized when prescription is issued
Distribution Between Registrants	DEA Form 222	Invoices	Invoices
Theft or Significant Loss	Report and complete DEA Form 106	Report and complete DEA Form 106	Report and complete DEA Form 106

Note: Keep all controlled substance records for two (2) years.

Exceptions: Faxed C-II prescriptions are valid for home infusion, long-term care, and hospice patients. Verbal C-II prescriptions are valid in emergencies, as long as the prescribing practitioner provides the pharmacy with a signed hardcopy within seven (7) days. * Where authorized by state law.

DRUG ADDICTION TREATMENT ACT OF 2000 (DATA 2000)

✓ Allows prescribers to obtain a waiver so they can prescribe Schedule III, IV, and V controlled substances for the treatment of opioid addiction outside of a registered narcotic treatment facility.

✓ Does NOT permit the prescribing of Schedule II controlled substances (i.e., methadone) for the treatment of opioid addiction outside of a registered narcotic treatment facility.

✓ Prescribers who have obtained the waiver possess a second DEA number that begins with the letter X.

METHADONE DISPENSING RESTRICTIONS

Only registered narcotic treatment facilities can dispense Schedule II controlled substances (methadone) for the treatment of opioid addiction. These facilities must complete a DEA Form 363 to apply for DEA registration.

DISPENSING METHADONE FROM A PHARMACY

⇨Dispensing methadone for the treatment of **pain** is **permitted**.
⇨Dispensing methadone for the treatment of **addiction** is **prohibited**.

PROFESSIONALS WITH PRESCRIBING AUTHORITY

There are two categories of prescribing authority: full authority and limited authority. Four types of healthcare practitioners have full prescribing authority: licensed physicians, dentists, podiatrists, and veterinarians. These practitioners can prescribe any medication **within their scope of practice**. This means veterinarians cannot prescribe medication for humans, dentists cannot prescribe medication for conditions of the eye, etc. Below, we have illustrated the four types of healthcare professionals and the respective academic degrees that confer full prescribing authority. Keep in mind, in addition to meeting the educational requirements, these practitioners must also obtain a license by passing certain board examinations and meeting other regulatory requirements.

PRACTITIONERS WITH <u>FULL</u> PRESCRIBING AUTHORITY

PHYSICIANS
Doctor of Medicine (MD)
Doctor of Osteopathic Medicine (DO)

PODIATRISTS
Doctor of Podiatric Medicine (DPM)

DENTISTS
Doctor of Dental Medicine (DMD)
Doctor of Dental Surgery (DDS)

VETERINARIANS
Doctor of Veterinary Medicine (DVM)

Optometrists and mid-level practitioners have limited prescribing authority. Depending on the state in which they practice, optometrists have certain restrictions and/or limitations regarding what they can prescribe, especially when it comes to controlled substances. The same is true for mid-level practitioners, such as physician assistants and nurse practitioners. Additionally, mid-level practitioners can only prescribe specific medications as outlined in a signed, written agreement with their supervising physician. A licensed physician must approve every prescription written by a mid-level practitioner.

PRACTITIONERS WITH <u>LIMITED</u> PRESCRIBING AUTHORITY

OPTOMETRISTS
Doctor of Optometry (OD)

MID-LEVEL PRACTITIONERS
Physician Assistant (PA)
Nurse Practitioner (NP)

Note: Some states grant limited prescribing authority to additional groups of qualified healthcare professionals, such as certified nurse midwives, certified registered nurse anesthetists, chiropractors, and registered pharmacists.

DEA NUMBER VERIFICATION

Sample DEA#: MH4836726

A prescriber cannot legally issue a controlled substance prescription unless he/she possesses a valid DEA registration number, which must appear on the face of every controlled substance prescription they issue. You may want to verify a DEA number before dispensing a controlled substance, especially if forgery is suspected. DEA numbers are composed of 2 letters followed by 7 numbers. First, we will review the letters.

THE 1ST LETTER: Functions to identify the type of practitioner/registrant.
- A, B, or F for physicians, dentists, veterinarians, hospitals, and pharmacies.
- M for mid-level practitioners.
- P or R for manufacturers, distributors, researchers, and narcotic treatment programs.

> **Note:** Practitioners with a waiver to prescribe buprenorphine (e.g., Subutex® and Suboxone®) for the treatment of opioid addiction outside of a narcotic treatment facility have a second DEA number, which begins with the letter X.

THE 2ND LETTER: Matches the first letter of the prescriber's last name or the first letter of the business name.

Once the letters have been verified, proceed to the 4-step process for the verifying the numerical portion of a DEA number, which is outlined below.

THE 4-STEP PROCESS FOR VERIFYING THE NUMERICAL PORTION OF A DEA NUMBER:

---STEP 1---
Add the 1st, 3rd, and 5th digits of the DEA number.

---STEP 2---
Add the 2nd, 4th, and 6th digits of the DEA number and multiply the sum by 2.

> **Note:** Remember to multiply the correct set of numbers by 2. Many students mistakenly multiply the sum of the 1st, 3rd, and 5th digits by 2 and get the wrong answer.

---STEP 3---
Add your answers from STEP 1 and STEP 2.

---STEP 4---
The sum obtained in STEP 3 will be a 2-digit number. If the DEA number is legitimate, then the second digit of this 2-digit number will match the 7th and final digit (known as the "check digit") of the DEA number.

➲ TRY IT YOURSELF! ➲

Analyze the sample DEA# shown at the top of this page. You should conclude that the number is valid. Once finished, continue to the "practice problem" shown on the following page.

FEDERAL GOVERNMENT PRACTITIONER EXEMPTION 21 CFR § 1301.23

Practitioners who are officials of the US Army, Navy, Marines, Air Force, Coast Guard, Public Health Service, or Bureau of Prisons are not required to register with the DEA to prescribe controlled substances unless they work in private practice. In place of the DEA number, these practitioners must indicate their branch of service or the agency in which they serve and their service identification number (e.g., Army 123-45-6789).

DEA NUMBER VERIFICATION
PRACTICE PROBLEM

VERIFY THE DEA NUMBER DISPLAYED BELOW.

John Smith, MD
DEA # FS8524616

SOLUTION

THE 1ST LETTER: The registrant is a physician (MD), so the first letter must be "A, B, or F."
THE 2ND LETTER: The prescriber's last name is Smith, so the second letter must be "S."

--STEP 1--
Add the 1st, 3rd, and 5th digits of the DEA number.

⇨ The sum of the 1st, 3rd, and 5th numbers (8 + 2 + 6) is 16.

--STEP 2--
Add the 2nd, 4th, and 6th digits of the DEA number and multiply the sum by 2.

⇨ The sum of the 2nd, 4th, and 6th numbers (5 + 4 + 1) is 10, and 10 x 2 = 20.

Note: Remember to multiply the correct set of numbers by 2. Many students mistakenly multiply the sum of the 1st, 3rd, and 5th digits by 2 and get the wrong answer.

--STEP 3--
Add your answers from STEP 1 and STEP 2.

⇨ The sum of 16 and 20 is 36.

--STEP 4--
Verify that the final digit of your answer from STEP 3 matches the check digit of the DEA number.

⇨ The final digit of the answer from STEP 3 is the number 6, which matches the check digit of the DEA number.

✔

**ACCORDING TO THE ANALYSIS OUTLINED ABOVE,
THIS DEA NUMBER APPEARS TO BE LEGITIMATE.**

Note: The Drug Addiction Treatment Act of 2000 (DATA 2000) requires prescribers to include their special DEA number (which begins with the letter X) on buprenorphine prescriptions issued for the treatment of opioid addiction. For example, Dr. John Smith's special DEA number (if he had one) would look like this: XS8524616.

INSTITUTIONAL DEA NUMBERS

When acting in the usual course of employment, practitioners and residents working for an institution (e.g., hospital) may prescribe controlled substances using the institution's DEA number. Institutions must assign an internal code number to each practitioner. The practitioner must append this code to the end of the institution's DEA number when writing prescriptions for controlled substances. See below for an example.

INSTITUTION'S DEA NUMBER   PRACTITIONER'S INTERNAL CODE
⇩   ⇩
AB8524616 - 1234

Each institution must keep a list of practitioners and their assigned internal codes to enable other DEA registrants, such as pharmacies, to contact the institution and verify that a particular practitioner is authorized to prescribe controlled substances.

ADDITIONAL DETAILS REGARDING DEA NUMBERS

Unlike the National Provider Identifier (NPI) number, which HIPAA requires all prescribers to have, not every prescriber must have a DEA number. Only practitioners who prescribe controlled substances are required to have a DEA number, which can be obtained by registering with the Drug Enforcement Administration. Any entity that handles controlled substances is also required to register with the DEA, including drug manufacturers, distributors, research labs, hospitals, and pharmacies.

PSEUDOEPHEDRINE

The law (Combat Methamphetamine Epidemic Act of 2005) imposes regulations on the over the counter sale of solid dosage forms (including gel caps) containing pseudoephedrine, ephedrine, or phenylpropanolamine. These substances are precursors to either amphetamine or methamphetamine.

PRECURSOR		POTENTIAL END PRODUCT
Pseudoephedrine	⇨	Methamphetamine
Ephedrine	⇨	Methamphetamine
Phenylpropanolamine	⇨	Amphetamine

BEFORE PURCHASING, THE CUSTOMER MUST FURNISH PHOTO ID

OTC PURCHASE LIMITS
- Daily Limit: 3.6 grams/day per customer
- Monthly Limit: 9 grams/month per customer

Per 21 CFR § 844(a), a maximum of 7.5 grams of the monthly 9-gram limit can be obtained by mail

PHARMACY RECORDKEEPING REQUIREMENTS
- Product name & quantity sold
- Name, address, & signature of purchaser
- Date & time of sale

Records must be maintained for at least 2 years

LIMITS DO NOT APPLY WHEN OBTAINED BY PRESCRIPTION

PHARMACY STORAGE REQUIREMENT
Solid dosage forms (including gel caps) that contain pseudoephedrine, ephedrine, or phenylpropanolamine must be stored behind the pharmacy counter or in a locked cabinet away from customers.

MANUFACTURER PACKAGING REQUIREMENT
Solid dosage forms (including gel caps) that contain pseudoephedrine, ephedrine, or phenylpropanolamine must be packaged in blister packs (see illustration below).

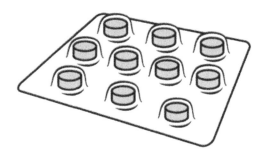

RESTRICTED DRUG PROGRAMS

As we know, medications have potential benefits (the intended therapeutic effect) and risks (side effects). Drugs that cause more harm than good typically do not reach the market, or, if they have already entered the market, are withdrawn once the harm is recognized (e.g., Vioxx®). Some medications are capable of causing great harm and yet provide tremendous benefit for certain patients. This is where restricted drug programs come into play. Pursuant to the FDA Amendments Act of 2007, the FDA can require manufacturers to comply with programs that help manage the risks associated with the use of certain drugs. These programs are also referred to as "Risk Evaluation and Mitigation Strategies" (REMS). Over 100 drugs are associated with a REMS program. The most well-known REMS programs are iPLEDGE™, THALOMID REMS™, T.I.P.S., and Clozaril® National Registry. In this section of the study guide, we review the basic elements of each of these four programs.

iPLEDGE™
Isotretinoin is effective in the treatment of severe acne; however, the use of isotretinoin during pregnancy is associated with severe birth defects. Among other requirements, iPLEDGE™ primarily mitigates this risk by:

1) Ensuring that patients who begin isotretinoin therapy are not pregnant
2) Preventing pregnancy in patients who receive isotretinoin

OTHER IMPORTANT POINTS:
✓ Isotretinoin prescriptions are limited to a 30-day supply.
✓ Isotretinoin brand name formulations include Absorbica®, Accutane®, Amnesteem®, Claravis®, Myorisan®, Sotret®, and Zenatane®.

THALOMID REMS™ (formerly known as S.T.E.P.S.®)
Thalomid® (thalidomide) is effective in the treatment of multiple myeloma and erythema nodosum leprosum; however, the use of thalidomide during pregnancy is associated with severe birth defects (e.g. "The Thalidomide Tragedy"). Among other requirements, THALOMID REMS™ primarily mitigates this risk by:

1) Ensuring that patients who begin thalidomide therapy are not pregnant
2) Preventing pregnancy in patients who receive thalidomide

OTHER IMPORTANT POINTS:
✓ Thalidomide prescriptions are limited to a 28-day supply with no refills or telephone prescriptions.
✓ The THALOMID REMS™ program was previously known as S.T.E.P.S.® (System for Thalidomide Education and Prescribing Safety).

T.I.P.S.
T.I.P.S. stands for "Tikosyn® In Pharmacy System." Tikosyn® (dofetilide) is used to induce and maintain normal cardiac sinus rhythm in highly symptomatic patients with atrial fibrillation or atrial flutter; however, the use of dofetilide is associated with potentially fatal ventricular arrhythmias, especially in patients who are starting or re-starting the drug. T.I.P.S. mitigates this risk by:

1) Communicating the risk of cardiac arrhythmias associated with Tikosyn® (dofetilide)
2) Requiring patients who receive Tikosyn® (dofetilide) to be admitted to a facility for medical monitoring for at least three (3) days when starting or re-starting therapy

Clozaril® National Registry

Clozaril® (clozapine) is effective in the treatment of various psychiatric disorders (e.g. schizophrenia, bipolar disorder); however, the use of clozapine is associated with potentially fatal agranulocytosis (suppression of white blood cell production). Clozaril® National Registry mitigates this risk by:

1) Requiring WBC count to be recorded in the Clozaril® National Registry **weekly for the first six (6) months** of therapy and then periodically thereafter
2) Limiting the amount of the drug pharmacies can dispense to a quantity sufficient only to treat the patient until their next scheduled lab work (e.g. a 7-day supply every week for the first six (6) months)

> **Note:** Sometimes this REMS program is referred to as the "No Blood, No Drug Program."

EACH REMS PROGRAM IS UNIQUE

Some REMS programs are so simple that you might not even realize they exist. A great example is Dulera® (mometasone/formoterol), for which the REMS program only imposes one (1) requirement – the manufacturer must communicate to healthcare providers the increased risk of asthma-related death associated with the use of long-acting beta agonists (such as formoterol found in Dulera®). On the other end of the spectrum, we see programs like the ones discussed in this section (iPLEDGE™, Thalomid REMS™, T.I.P.S., and Clozaril® National Registry) that impose tougher rules and require participation by multiple parties (e.g., the doctor, the patient, and/or the pharmacy). Each REMS program is unique.

OTHER IMPORTANT POINTS REGARDING REMS PROGRAMS

✓ Manufacturers may implement a REMS program for a drug in the absence of an FDA requirement to do so.
✓ The consequence for a manufacturer that fails to comply with a REMS program is a fine of at least $250,000 per incident.

MANUFACTURER DRUG PACKAGE LABELING

This section pertains to stock bottle labeling for prescription drugs. The labeling on a stock container provides information for the pharmacist regarding not only the contents but also dosage and use information for safe and effective prescribing. From a pharmacy perspective, the most important elements of labeling are 1) the manufacturer's drug package label, which is the label affixed to the stock bottle or container, and 2) the package insert, also commonly referred to as the prescribing information. The exam may test your ability to locate certain information. For instance, where can you find the expiration date? Where can you find information on dosage and administration? Study the outline below to familiarize yourself with the categories of information that appear on the manufacturer's drug package label.

REQUIRED INFORMATION FOR A MANUFACTURER'S DRUG PACKAGE LABEL

- Brand drug name*
- Generic drug name
- Name and location of the manufacturer, packer, or distributor
- Drug strength or concentration
- Type of dosage form
- Total weight, volume, or number of dosage units contained in the package
- The statement "Caution: federal law prohibits dispensing without a prescription" or "Rx Only"

- A statement that refers individuals to the prescribing information (the package insert) for more information
- Storage instructions
- National Drug Code (NDC number) with barcode**
- Expiration date
- Lot number
- A symbol representing the controlled substance schedule in which the drug is listed (i.e., CII, CIII, CIV, or CV) ***

*For brand name products only. Does not apply to generics.
**NDC numbers are recommended, but not required.
***For controlled substances only.

Note: The FDA recommends that manufacturers obtain and include an NDC number on the drug package label, but this is not a requirement. Manufacturers are aware that pharmacies rely heavily on NDC numbers when purchasing medications and maintaining inventory records, so it is in the manufacturers' best interest to include an NDC number on the label. Only in very rare cases will you see a drug package label without an NDC number.

EXAMPLE
MANUFACTURER DRUG PACKAGE LABEL

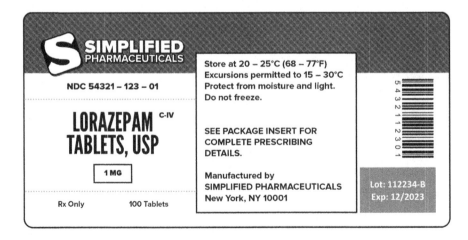

REQUIRED INFORMATION FOR A PACKAGE INSERT (PRESCRIBING INFORMATION)

Most manufacturers fold the package insert into a small square and glue it to the cap on the stock prescription bottle. The information on the package insert must be unbiased and scientific. The information in the package insert is for healthcare professionals, not patients or consumers. The FDA requires certain information to appear on a package insert. In 2001, the requirements changed. The information included on the package insert will depend on when the drug received FDA-approval. Memorizing all of this information is not necessary. The important thing is that you have a general idea about where to find specific information.

Information Category Requirements for Drugs Approved Before June 30, 2001:

- Description
- Clinical Pharmacology
- Indications and Usage
- Contraindications
- Warnings
- Precautions
- Adverse Reactions

- Drug Abuse and Dependence**
- Overdosage
- Dosage and Administration
- How Supplied
- Animal Pharmacology/Toxicology
- Clinical Studies
- References

* Drugs approved by the FDA prior to 6/30/2001 are not required to conform to the updated labeling requirements outlined below, but conformance is recommended/encouraged.

**Sections that clearly do not apply need not be included on the package insert. For instance, the section titled "Drug Abuse and Dependence" need not appear on the package insert of a non-controlled substance medication.

Information Category Requirements for Drugs Approved on or After June 30, 2001:

- Boxed Warning
- Indications and Usage
- Dosage and Administration
- Dosage Forms and Strengths
- Contraindications
- Warnings and Precautions
- Adverse Reactions
- Drug Interactions
- Use in Specific Populations

- Drug Abuse and Dependence
- Overdosage
- Description
- Clinical Pharmacology
- Nonclinical Toxicology
- Clinical Studies
- References
- How Supplied/Storage & Handling
- Patient Counseling Information

OVER THE COUNTER DRUG PACKAGE LABELING

You also need to be familiar with the different categories of information found on an over the counter (OTC) drug package label. As we have mentioned in other sections, OTC medications, unlike prescription medications, are therapeutic agents that customers can purchase without a prescription. Examples include Tums®, Tylenol®, Motrin®, Mucinex®, Prilosec®, and Prevacid®. For our list of the top 50 OTC drugs, see pages 70-71.

To get the most out of reviewing this section, we recommend that you retrieve an OTC medication from your drug cabinet at home. If you do not have any OTC medication, then can use the back of your tube of fluoride toothpaste. It will be close enough. Study the label and compare it to the outline below.

REQUIRED INFORMATION FOR AN OTC DRUG PACKAGE LABEL

- Drug Facts
    - Active Ingredient(s) and strength or concentration per dosage unit.
    - Purpose(s).
- Uses
    - A list of the approved indications/uses.
- Warnings
    - Statements regarding allergies, use in pregnancy and breast-feeding, overdose, drug interactions, age-related warnings, and when to consult a doctor or pharmacist. The statement, "Keep out of reach of children."
- Directions
    - Specific instructions based on age, recommended dose, frequency of dosing, and maximum daily dose. For example, the directions for Tylenol® Extra Strength may say, "Adults and children age 12 years and older: take 1 – 2 tablets up to every 6 hours while symptoms last. Do not exceed 6 tablets in 24 hours, unless directed by a doctor.
- Other Information
    - Storage requirements.
    - Details regarding electrolyte content (if applicable).
- Inactive Ingredients
    - List of ingredients that do not affect therapeutic action, such as flavoring agents, colorants, and preservatives.
- Contact Information
    - Company name, location, and phone number of the manufacturer.
- Statement regarding the integrity of the tamper-evident packaging, such as "Do not use if safety seal is broken or missing" *
- Expiration date and lot number**

* The FDA requires tamper-evident packaging for most OTC medications. This requirement was established after the 1982 Chicago Tylenol Murders, where someone obtained Tylenol, then laced the capsules with cyanide and returned the bottles to the shelf, leading to the death of seven people.

** If you are following along with a tube of fluoride toothpaste, the expiration date and lot number can be hard to see. It is usually stamped into the crimped end of the tube.

REPACKAGING MEDICATIONS

Many regulations address drug packaging and labeling (e.g., FDA Compliance Policy Guideline CPG Sec 430-100). From a regulatory point of view, the easiest thing to do is leave medications in the stock bottle (as supplied by the manufacturer) until the time of dispensing; however, there are undeniable benefits to repackaging. These benefits mainly apply to hospitals and other inpatient facilities. By transferring medications to unit-dose (single dose) packages, each dose obtains its own identifying label, helping inpatient facilities ensure the right drug is going to the right patient. Additionally, unit-dose packaging protects individual doses from the moisture and contamination. Consequently, the pharmacy can retrieve and re-dispense unused doses, thereby reducing waste.

For the reasons described above, it is common for pharmacies, particularly in a hospital setting, to repackage medications. The process of repackaging is simple and merely involves transferring individual doses (e.g., one tablet or capsule, or one or two teaspoons of a liquid) from a medication stock bottle into smaller, single-use packages. Once the pharmacy transfers a medication from its original stock bottle into unit-dose packages, the stability of the drug falls into question. Will the drug be stable in this new environment? The repackaging material may accelerate the expiration of the drug. Pharmacies can perform stability tests, but these tests can be expensive and, in most cases, impractical. As an alternative, the FDA suggests assigning a beyond-use date (BUD) equal to six (6) months, provided this does not exceed 25% of the time remaining between the date of repackaging and the manufacturer-assigned expiration date printed on the label of the stock bottle.

Pharmacies can only use the 6-month beyond-use date shortcut for nonsterile liquid and solid dosage forms. In addition, the product must come from a previously unopened stock bottle, and the entire contents of the stock bottle must be repackaged in one operation. The repackaging process and subsequent storage of the product must comply with the manufacturer specifications for storage and handling (typically room temperature with relative humidity 75% or less). This information can be located in the package insert of any given drug. Pharmacy technicians can only repackage medications under the direct supervision of a licensed pharmacist, and most states require maintenance of a repackaging log that documents the details of repackaging (e.g., date repackaged, name of person repackaging). Take note that the FDA prohibits the repackaging of nitroglycerin sublingual tablets and other products with known stability issues.

SUMMARY OF UNIT-DOSE PACKAGE LABEL REQUIREMENTS

- Drug name & strength
- Beyond-use date
- Lot number
- Name and location of repackager
- A statement indicating special dosage form characteristics, if applicable (e.g., chewable, extended release)
- NDC number (recommended, not required)
- If greater than one, the number of unit doses contained in each package
- For controlled substances, the statement "Warning: May be habit forming" along with the controlled substance symbol (e.g., C-II, C-III, C-IV, or C-V)
- For prescription drugs, "Rx Only" or a similar statement

FDA RECALLS

A recall is the voluntary removal (or correction) of a product that violates the United States Federal Food, Drug, and Cosmetic Act. Typically, a recall is required when an FDA-regulated product is found to be "adulterated" or "misbranded." To understand the difference between adulteration and misbranding, see below.

ADULTERATED vs. MISBRANDED

ADULTERATED	MISBRANDED
Problem(s) with the **product**, such as the:	Problem(s) with the **labeling**, such as:
✓ Strength of the product.	✓ False information.
✓ Quality of the product.	✓ Misleading information.
✓ Purity of the product.	✓ Insufficient information.

If an FDA-regulated product, such as a drug, medical device, or dietary supplement, is found to pose a serious risk to the health of consumers (or if it is determined that consumers have been deceived), and the product is not voluntarily recalled by the manufacturer, then the FDA may issue a recall in the interest of protecting the public health and welfare. Pharmacies commonly receive product recall notifications as they are announced. Pharmacy personnel must respond quickly to remove any recalled items to prevent or minimize consumer exposure.

FDA RECALL CLASSIFICATIONS

FDA-assigned recall classifications indicate the degree of risk associated with the use of the recalled product.

CLASS I RECALL
The use of (or exposure to) the affected product could cause serious adverse health consequences or death.

CLASS II RECALL
The use of (or exposure to) the affected product could cause temporary or medically reversible adverse health consequences, and the likelihood of serious adverse health consequences is remote.

CLASS III RECALL
The use of (or exposure to) the affected product is unlikely to cause adverse health consequences.

REVIEW QUESTION

Which is the most serious type of FDA recall?

A. Class I Recall
B. Class II Recall
C. Class III Recall
D. Red Alert Recall

Answer: A. Class I Recall

PATIENT SAFETY AND QUALITY ASSURANCE

LOOK-ALIKE/SOUND-ALIKE MEDICATIONS

Each health care organization seeking to satisfy the requirements of the National Patient Safety Goals (a set of requirements that are part of the Joint Commission accreditation* process) must develop a look-alike/sound-alike medication list for their organization. See below for an example of a look-alike/sound-alike medication list:

Aciphex & Aricept	Durasal & Durezol	Oracea & Orencia
Advair & Advicor	Fioricet & Fiorinal	Oxycodone & Oxycontin
Alprazolam & Lorazepam	Flonase & Flovent	Patanol & Platinol
Amlodipine & Amiloride	Fomepizole & Omeprazole	Pentobarbital & Phenobarbital
Benadryl & Benazepril	Glyburide & Glipizide	Prograf & Prozac
Bupropion & Buspirone	Guaifenesin & Guanfacine	Quinine & Quinidine
Celebrex & Celexa**	Hydralazine & Hydroxyzine**	Risperidone & Ropinirole
Celebrex & Cerebyx	Kapidex & Casodex	Sitagliptin & Sumatriptan
Clomiphene & Clomipramine	Keppra & Keflex	Tiagabine & Tizanidine
Clonidine & Klonopin**	Lamictal & Lamisil	Tramadol & Trazadone**
Clozaril & Colazal	Lunesta & Neulasta	Vinblastine & Vincristine**
Codeine & Lodine	Metformin & Metronidazole	Wellbutrin SR & Wellbutrin XL
Diprivan & Ditropan	Mirapex & Miralax	Zantac & Zyrtec
Dobutamine & Dopamine	Misoprostol & Mifepristone	

*Joint Commission accreditation is intended to be a mark of high-quality care. Health care organizations usually seek Joint Commission accreditation because, in many states, it is a precondition to receiving Medicare and Medicaid payments.
**These are some of the most notorious look-alike/sound-alike names.

HIGH-ALERT MEDICATIONS

High-alert (or "high-risk") medications are drugs with a high likelihood of causing serious harm, especially when used improperly. The Joint Commission (a nonprofit organization that accredits health care organizations) requires each hospital to develop their own list of medications that they consider to be in the high-risk category. As a result, the medications that are considered high-risk may vary from one institution to another. See below for the drugs/drug classes that usually appear on an institution's high-alert medication list.

ANTICOAGULANTS (e.g., warfarin, heparin, enoxaparin, apixaban, rivaroxaban, dabigatran)
Anticoagulants are used to treat and prevent blood clots, but they can cause potentially fatal bleeding if too much is administered.

METHOTREXATE
Methotrexate is a cancer chemotherapeutic agent; however, the oral tablet version of methotrexate is commonly prescribed for less serious conditions involving inflammation, such as arthritis, in doses ≤ 30 mg once per week. If taken more frequently or in higher doses (for conditions other than cancer), patient harm up to and including death can occur.

NEUROMUSCULAR BLOCKERS (e.g., rocuronium, succinylcholine, pancuronium)
Neuromuscular blockers are commonly used to stop breathing to allow for mechanical ventilation. These drugs are considered to be high-risk since they interfere with the ability to breathe.

OPIOIDS (e.g., fentanyl, methadone, morphine, hydrocodone, oxycodone)
Opioids are used to treat pain, but they have the potential to cause fatal respiratory depression at high doses.

INSULIN (e.g., Humulin® R, Novolin® R, Humalog®, NovoLog®, Apidra®, Lantus®, Levemir®)
Insulin decreases blood sugar by increasing cellular utilization of glucose, which has a therapeutic effect for patients with diabetes, but too much insulin can cause hypoglycemia*. In severe cases, hypoglycemia can be fatal. Insulin U-500, which is five times more concentrated than most insulin preparations, receives special emphasis.

*Hypoglycemia means low blood sugar. Symptoms of hypoglycemia include dizziness, confusion, shakiness, sweating, and heart palpitations.

ERROR PREVENTION STRATEGIES

1) USE TALL MAN LETTERING

Tall man lettering is a way to emphasize the difference in drug names that otherwise look similar. For instance, Hydroxyzine and Hydralazine are two drug names that, at first glance, look quite similar. When you use tall man lettering (HydrOXYzine and HydrALAZINE), the differences in spelling are emphasized, thus reducing the chance that one will be misinterpreted as the other.

Below is a modified list from FDA.gov that demonstrates the use of tall man lettering for look-alike/sound-alike drugs:

AcetaHEXAMIDE	⇔	AcetaZOLAMIDE
BuPROPion	⇔	BusPIRone
ChlorproMAZINE	⇔	ChlorproPAMIDE
ClomiPHENE	⇔	ClomiPRAMINE
CycloSPORINE	⇔	CycloSERINE
DAUNOrubicin	⇔	DOXOrubicin
DimenhyDRINATE	⇔	DiphenhydrAMINE
DOBUTamine	⇔	DOPamine
HydrALAZINE	⇔	HydrOXYzine
MethylPREDNISolone	⇔	MethylTESTOSTERone
NiCARdipine	⇔	NIFEdipine
PredniSONE	⇔	PrednisoLONE
risperiDONE	⇔	rOPINIRole
SulfADIAZINE	⇔	SulfiSOXAZOLE
TOLAZamide	⇔	TOLBUTamide
VinBLAStine	⇔	VinCRIStine

2) SEPARATE INVENTORY

A popular method for preventing medication dispensing errors is separating inventory. When medications are organized alphabetically, it is common to have drugs with very similar names stored right next to each other on the shelf (e.g., Isosorbide Mononitrate & Isosorbide Dinitrate or Metoprolol Tartrate & Metoprolol Succinate). The advantages of separating medications that have similar names are: #1 There is less of a chance that the bottles will get mixed up during storage, and #2 The person filling the prescription is forced to stop and think rather than quickly reach for the first drug that appears to be correct.

3) USE LEADING ZEROS

Leading zeros help to ensure accurate translation of numbers less than 1. By omitting a leading zero, you run the risk of causing the patient to receive a dose many times higher than the intended dose. This can be a fatal mistake.

Acceptable: 0.1, 0.005, 0.02, 0.99
Unacceptable: .1, .005, .02, .99

What is the difference between .99 and 0.99?
.99 could easily be misinterpreted as ninety-nine. Consider how detrimental it would be if a patient was supposed to get 0.99 grams of a drug, and they ended up getting 99 grams. One hundred times higher than the prescribed dose. Depending on the drug, an error this big could be fatal.

4) AVOID TRAILING ZEROS

While leading zeros can prevent fatal dispensing errors, trailing zeros can cause them. Imagine that a practitioner writes a prescription for Alprazolam 1 mg PO QID PRN anxiety, but when writing the prescription, the practitioner used a trailing zero (one milligram is written as "1.0 mg"). Therefore, the prescription looks like this:

Alprazolam 1.0 mg PO QID PRN anxiety

The decimal point between the number one and the trailing zero is barely visible! When reading this prescription, the technician and pharmacist could easily misinterpret the strength as ten (10) milligrams instead of one (1) milligram. This misinterpretation could lead to a fatal dispensing error. Never use trailing zeros. Write one as 1, not 1.0 or 1.00.

5) AVOID ERROR-PRONE ABBREVIATIONS

Another safety strategy is to avoid the use of error-prone abbreviations. Much like leading and trailing zeros, certain abbreviations can lead to dangerous misinterpretations. The FDA and ISMP* have teamed up in a campaign to eliminate the use of error-prone abbreviations. The list below summarizes the most common error-prone abbreviations. Generally, it is best to write out the instructions word for word and avoid abbreviations altogether.

ERROR-PRONE ABBREVIATION →	POTENTIAL MISINTERPRETATION
AD (right ear)	OD (right eye)
AS (left ear)	OS (left eye)
AU (both ears)	OU (both eyes)
OD (right eye)	AD (right ear)
OS (left eye)	AS (left ear)
OU (both eyes)	AU (both ears)
cc (cubic centimeters)	U (units)
HS (bedtime)	HS (half-strength) or HR (hour)
BT (bedtime)	BID (twice daily)
IU (international units)	IV (intravenous)
IN (intranasal)	IM (intramuscular)
QD or Q1D (daily)	QID (four times daily)
QOD (every other day)	QD (daily) or QID (four times daily)
OD (right eye)	QD (daily)
SC or SQ (subcutaneous)	5 Q ___ (five every...)
ss (one-half)	55 (fifty-five)
1/D (one per day)	TID (three times daily)
° (hours; e.g., 6° = 6 hours)	0 (zero; e.g., 60 = sixty)
UD (as directed)	Unit Dose
Per os (by mouth)	OS (left eye)

*The Institute for Safe Medication Practices (ISMP) is a nonprofit organization devoted to preventing medication errors and ensuring the safe use of medications.

6) READ BACK VERBAL PRESCRIPTIONS

In certain states (assuming company policy permits), certified pharmacy technicians can accept verbal prescriptions for non-controlled substances from a prescriber (or an agent of the prescriber) over the phone. If you have this privilege/responsibility, always remember to convert the verbal order to writing immediately, write legibly, and read the order back to the prescriber (or the agent of the prescriber) to verify that all of the information was communicated correctly. This is important because, as a good friend of mine says, "What is said is not always the same as what is heard."

7) PROMOTE PATIENT COUNSELING

Patient counseling is the final opportunity to catch a dispensing error before it ends up in the hands of the patient and causes harm. During a patient counseling session, the pharmacist will go over information like the brand and generic name of the medication, what the drug is used to treat, the dose prescribed, etc. Not only is this an opportunity for the patient to receive some basic education on the medicines they take, but it is also an opportunity to identify errors. For instance, let's say you drop-off a prescription for a blood pressure medication. When you go to pick up the medication, the pharmacist explains that the medication is used to treat bacterial infections and then asks you if you have an infection. You say, "No, I have high blood pressure." Disaster averted – the pharmacist realizes that this is a potential dispensing error and takes this opportunity to correct the error before it harms the patient. Even if the patient refuses counseling, at least go over the medication name(s) with them before they purchase the prescription(s).

8) USE BAR-CODE TECHNOLOGY

The use of bar-code technology has been proven to reduce dispensing error rates significantly. Bar-code technology can be implemented during various steps in the prescription filling and dispensing process, but the most common and impactful step where this technology can be applied is scanning the bar-code of the stock bottle after selecting the drug off of the shelf to verify the drug is correct prior to filling a prescription. Some institutions also use this technology to reduce nursing errors in medication administration (known as Bar-Code Medication Administration or "BCMA").

9) MATCHING NDCs

It is important for technicians and pharmacists to ensure that the NDC number of the drug used to fill a prescription is the same as the NDC number being used for billing the insurance. It is also important when filling a prescription from more than one stock bottle of medication to ensure that all stock bottles used to fill the prescription have matching NDC numbers. This helps ensure that the patient receives the correct medication, and the details of the insurance claim match the details of the specific product being dispensed.

10) COMPUTERIZED PHYSICIAN ORDER ENTRY (CPOE)

Prescribers issue medication orders* by sending them electronically directly to the pharmacy department of the healthcare facility. Since prescriptions sent by this method are typed, CPOE helps prevent errors that might occur from the misinterpretation of a prescriber's handwriting.

11) E-PRESCRIBING

Prescribers issue prescriptions* by sending them electronically directly to the patients' pharmacy of choice. Just like CPOE, e-prescribing helps reduce errors that might occur from the misinterpretation of a prescriber's handwriting.

*Medication orders and prescriptions are similar, but they have one distinct difference. Medication orders are issued for drugs that will be administered within a healthcare facility (e.g., a hospital); whereas, prescriptions are issued for drugs that will be used outside of a healthcare facility.

THE ROLE OF PHARMACY TECHNICIANS

What major activities fall under the scope of pharmacy practice?
- Interpreting, evaluating, and implementing prescriptions and medication orders.
- Compounding and dispensing prescriptions.
- Participating in the selection and administration of drugs and medical devices.
- Performing drug utilization reviews and evaluating the appropriateness and safety of new and existing drug therapies.
- Creating and maintaining patient medication profiles and pharmacy records.
- Counseling and advising patients and other healthcare professionals.
- Administering vaccinations and immunizations.
- Performing drug-related research.

WHAT IS THE PHARMACY TECHNICIAN'S PRIMARY ROLE?
To assist the pharmacist by completing technical tasks.

EXAMPLES OF TASKS THAT CAN BE COMPLETED BY A PHARMACY TECHNICIAN

- Creating and maintaining patient profiles and pharmacy records.
- Receiving written, faxed, and electronically transmitted prescriptions.
- Typing prescription labels.
- Filling prescription orders.
    - Retrieving drugs from stock.
    - Counting or measuring dosage units.
    - Placing dosage units in a container.
    - Affixing a label to the container.
    - Returning drugs to stock.
- Handling or delivering completed prescriptions.
- Alerting the pharmacist to situations that require professional judgment.
- Assisting the pharmacist in managing inventory (e.g., medications, vials/bottles, caps).
- Restocking inventory/placing new items on the shelves.
- Identifying and removing expired products from the inventory.
- Disposing of expired or contaminated products according to policies & procedures.
- Removing and returning recalled, discontinued, and overstocked items from the pharmacy's inventory.
- Maintaining the organization and cleanliness of the pharmacy and patient care areas.
- Maintaining the security of the prescription area.
    - Following procedures intended to prevent unauthorized individuals from entering the pharmacy (e.g., lock the doors, engage the security gate, and activate the alarm during the pharmacist's absence).
- Complying with rules and regulations related to the practice of pharmacy.

NOTE: A pharmacist must check all work completed by a pharmacy technician.

ISSUES REQUIRING PHARMACIST INTERVENTION

In recent years, the role of the pharmacy technician has expanded significantly. Nonetheless, there are still several tasks and issues that can only be addressed by a licensed pharmacist. Generally, these are situations that require some degree of professional judgment. See below for examples.

DRUG UTILIZATION REVIEW (DUR)

Only a pharmacist can complete a DUR (i.e., evaluate the appropriateness and safety of drug therapy). The purpose of the review is to identify and respond to potential and actual drug interactions, therapeutic duplications, incorrect dosages, drug allergies, potential cases of drug misuse, abuse, non-adherence (cases where the patients does not appear to be taking the medication as frequently as prescribed), and other medication-related issues requiring professional judgment for resolution.

EVALUATE THE LEGALITY OF A PRESCRIPTION

Evaluate prescriptions for authenticity and conformance with legal requirements.

THERAPEUTIC SUBSTITUTION DECISIONS

Whenever dispensing a medication other than what was originally prescribed (i.e., a generic substitute), a pharmacist must make the final decision regarding product selection.

OTC RECOMMENDATIONS

All requests for over the counter (OTC) drug recommendations must be deferred to a pharmacist. Pharmacy technicians cannot make OTC drug recommendations; however, if a patient merely asks where an OTC drug product is located in the business establishment, then a pharmacy technician can step in to help the patient locate the product.

PHARMACEUTICAL COUNSELING

Anytime a patient requests pharmaceutical counseling or has a question about a prescription drug (aside from basic information such as the name and strength of the drug), pharmacist intervention is required.

ADVICE REGARDING A MISSED DOSE

If a patient requests advice regarding what to do if they miss one or more scheduled doses of medication, then the pharmacist must step in to provide the patient with instructions regarding the most appropriate action.

RESPONSE TO AN ADVERSE DRUG EVENT (ADE)

A patient who complains or asks questions about a possible medication-related adverse event should speak directly to the pharmacist.

ADMINISTRATION OF IMMUNIZATIONS/POST-IMMUNIZATION FOLLOW-UP

In a pharmacy, only a pharmacist can administer immunizations. If a patient returns to the pharmacy due to an immunization-related adverse event, then the pharmacist should speak directly to the patient regarding the most appropriate action.

DISPENSING ERRORS

There are two general categories of event reporting:
#1 Internal (i.e., reporting dispensing errors in accordance with the pharmacy's quality assurance program).
#2 External (i.e., reporting errors and adverse events to the U.S. Food and Drug Administration).

Despite all of the efforts directed at error prevention, medication errors (e.g., prescribing errors made by physicians and dispensing errors made by pharmacies) still occur. See a list of common dispensing errors below.

- Incorrect patient*
- Incorrect drug
- Incorrect dose
- Incorrect dosage form
- Incorrect directions for use
- Incorrect duration of therapy
- Incorrect quantity
- Incorrect number of refills
- Incorrect preparation or storage

*When a patient mistakenly receives another patient's prescription, private information (known as "protected health information" or "PHI") the exposure of health information constitutes a breach of the Health Insurance Portability and Accountability Act (HIPAA), a law intended to protect the privacy of PHI. According to the HIPAA Breach Notification Rule, the pharmacy must respond by notifying the affected individual that her PHI was exposed.

When responding to any dispensing error, patient safety is the highest priority. Was the patient harmed as a result of the error? If so, the pharmacy must notify the patient's primary care provider and instruct the patient to seek medical attention immediately, depending on the seriousness of the situation. Regardless of whether the patient was harmed, the pharmacy must also document the error in accordance with the pharmacy's quality assurance program, which should be outlined in the policies and procedures. Most dispensing errors stem from a problem in the way the pharmacy operates, and addressing that problem could reduce the chance of a similar error happening again. Consequently, the report that is made to document the error should include a **root-cause analysis (RCA)** to identify the underlying cause of the error, as well as an action plan that outlines the steps that will be taken to fix the problem.

NEAR MISS ERRORS

Near misses are errors that occur but are caught by chance before they reach the patient. An example would be mistakenly filling a prescription for trazodone with tramadol. The patient arrives to pick up the prescription, but before purchasing it, he presents a new insurance card. While processing the prescription through the new insurance plan, you notice the error and correct the prescription before dispensing it to the patient. Even though the error never reached the patient, it is still helpful to document the near miss in accordance with the pharmacy's quality assurance program. By reporting near misses, the pharmacy can implement procedures to prevent a similar error from ever reaching a patient and causing harm.

MEDWATCH

Drug companies gain FDA approval for new drugs by conducting clinical trials. If trial data indicates their product is safe and effective, then FDA approval may be granted. After a drug is approved and enters the market, the FDA continues to gather safety information via "post-marketing safety surveillance," which is based on adverse event reports filed by patients, manufacturers, and healthcare professionals (e.g., physicians, pharmacists). Reporting an adverse drug event is voluntary. Even though adverse event reporting is not legally required, the FDA encourages healthcare professionals to report serious adverse events to help improve drug safety. Reports can lead to changes in product labeling, changes in recommendations for monitoring, product recalls, or market withdrawals. For example, Vioxx® (rofecoxib) was withdrawn from the market when data from post-marketing safety surveillance revealed an association between its use and an increase in the risk of cardiovascular events (e.g., heart attacks, strokes).

Reports on adverse events, medication errors, and product integrity problems (i.e., concerns regarding the safety, quality, performance, or authenticity of a drug product or medical device) can be filed through the FDA's MedWatch program (available at <https://www.fda.gov/medwatch>). MedWatch is appropriate for filing reports regarding prescription drugs, over the counter drugs, biologics, medical devices, special nutritional products, foods, and cosmetics.

VAERS

Adverse events related to vaccines should be reported through the Vaccine Adverse Event Reporting System (VAERS; available at <https://vaers.hhs.gov/reportevent.html>)

HYGIENE AND CLEANING STANDARDS

PHARMACY PERSONNEL
- Wash hands before and after interacting with patients.
- Do not handle medication if you have an active, potentially contagious infection.
- Avoid touching medications directly with your hands.
- Use clean spatulas, counting trays, and/or measuring devices to handle medications.
- If direct handling of medication is unavoidable, then wash hands, and use a clean pair of medical gloves.
- Never consume food in the pharmacy.
- Always wear clean clothing in the pharmacy.

EQUIPMENT & FACILITIES
- Storage bins should be cleaned when visibly soiled.
- Counting trays should be cleaned at least once daily with 70% isopropyl alcohol.
- Medication storage areas (including refrigerators) cannot be used to store food or drinks.
- Crash carts or drug kits contaminated with bodily fluids must be disinfected (e.g., with diluted bleach).
- Automated dispensing machines and refrigerators designated for drug storage should be cleaned routinely (e.g., once monthly) and additionally as needed.
- Countertops should be cleaned with 70% isopropyl alcohol once daily and additionally as needed.
- Floors should be free of clutter and cleaned routinely.

KNOWLEDGE AREA #4
ORDER ENTRY AND PROCESSING

NONSTERILE COMPOUNDING

USP Chapter <795> Pharmaceutical Compounding–Nonsterile Preparations
Provides guidance on good compounding practices in preparing non-sterile compounded drug products.

Compounding is the creation of a personalized, *patient-specific* drug preparation that takes place when commercially available drug products fail to meet the needs of the patient. For instance, a patient unable to swallow pills may be in need of a medication only available commercially as an oral tablet. In this case, the pharmacy may be able to step in to prepare a customized dosage form for the patient (e.g., an oral liquid).

Compounding pharmacies must adhere to the following basic guidelines (among others):
- A compounded drug product cannot be a copy of a commercially available FDA-approved drug product.
- A compounded drug product cannot contain any ingredient that has been deemed unsafe or ineffective.
- Products can only be compounded after receiving an individual, patient-specific prescription order (or in anticipation of receiving such an order, provided that an established prescribing pattern exists).

NOTEWORTHY REQUIREMENTS *of* USP CHAPTER <795>
- Always use purified water when water is part of the formulation.
- Rotate stock to ensure the oldest ingredients are used first.
- Handle and store ingredients/compounded preparations in a way to prevent contamination.
- Store ingredients/compounded preparations in a way to facilitate cleaning and inspection.
- Locate equipment in a way to prevent contamination and permit the use, maintenance, and cleaning.
- Routinely inspect and calibrate (if applicable) equipment to ensure proper function.
- Inspect equipment before using it.
- Clean equipment after using it.
- Store ingredients/compounded preparations under the proper conditions (e.g., temperature, humidity).
- Appropriately label all compounded preparations.
- If transferring an ingredient to a new container, ensure the integrity of the new container is at least as good as the original container.
- If transferring an ingredient to a new container, label the new container with the name of the ingredient, name of the supplier, lot number, transfer date, and expiration date.
- Use the appropriate equipment (proper design and size, and will not react with, absorb, disintegrate, dissolve, or leach into the compounded product).
- Meticulously clean equipment before re-using to compound different drugs.
- Label compounded preparations appropriately (including generic name, quantity or concentration of each active ingredient, BUD, storage and handling instructions, and assigned prescription number).

MASTER FORMULATION RECORD

When compounding a prescription, a **Master Formulation Record (MFR)** must be followed unless the instructions for compounding are provided directly on the manufacturer's label (e.g., as when reconstituting certain oral antibiotic suspensions). An MFR for compounding is conceptually similar to a recipe used in cooking. The MFR provides detailed instructions, including a list of ingredients and quantities, calculations, needed equipment, instructions for mixing, stability data, labeling information, requirements for packaging and storage, and quality control procedures.

COMPOUNDING RECORD

Each time a prescription is compounded, the details must be documented in the **compounding record (CR)**. For example, the names, sources, lot numbers, and expiration dates of all ingredients, the total quantity compounded, the names of the personnel who compounded, checked, and approved the final product, the date of compounding, the assigned prescription number, the beyond-use date, a copy of the label, and any quality control results/notes. Additionally, if a patient ever reported any adverse drug reactions in connection with a compounded prescription, this would also have to be documented in the CR.

BEYOND-USE DATES

A beyond-use date is a date after which a compounded medication should not be used. Beyond-use dates are typically short (i.e., days, weeks, or months) compared to expiration dates, which are usually one or more years. It is important to recognize that a "beyond-use date" and an "expiration date" are **not** the same thing. Manufacturers assign expiration dates to manufactured products; whereas, beyond-use dates are assigned to compounded and repackaged drug products.

Each ingredient in a compounded preparation has its own manufacturer-assigned expiration date, but the final compounded preparation has characteristics that are often different from the characteristics of any individual ingredient – for instance, the viscosity, the water content, and the preservative concentrations. Additionally, the container in which the final compounded preparation is stored is inevitably different from the original ingredient storage containers. Over time, unpredictable chemical reactions may occur, ultimately affecting the strength, quality, purity, and stability of the final compounded preparation. For that reason, it is necessary to determine a reasonable time through which we can be confident that the final compounded preparation will maintain the expected level of strength, quality, purity, and stability – the "beyond-use date."

Beyond-use dates also apply to opened vials containing sterile medication for injection (e.g., insulin, vitamin B12 injection solution). As with any other medication, a manufacturer assigns an expiration date for each vial and communicates this information to the pharmacy by stamping the expiration date on the vial label. This represents the manufacturer's guarantee that the contents of the container will be sterile, effective, and otherwise safe until the expiration date, provided that the medication is stored in compliance with the conditions specified on the label. The instant the vial is opened, the expiration date no longer applies because once opened, some bacteria will inevitably enter the vial and begin to multiply. The only question is, at what point after opening a vial of the sterile medication does the medication become unusable?

Unless the vial says "multi-dose" on the label, assume single use only. For single-use vials, we must discard any remaining content after initial use. The reason being, single-use vials do **not** contain preservatives to protect the contents from bacterial proliferation, and, as previously mentioned, some bacteria will infiltrate an open vial and multiply, even when employing the principles of aseptic technique. Multi-dose vials do contain preservatives. For that reason, disposal of unused portions of medication is not necessary; however, preservatives have their limits. Unless specified otherwise in the labeling, multi-dose vials (e.g., vials of insulin) can be assumed to have a BUD of 28 days after initial use.

MAXIMUM BEYOND-USE DATE (BUD) FOR NONSTERILE COMPOUNDED PRODUCTS*

Contains no water ("nonaqueous")	6 months
Topical/dermal or mucosal liquid that contains water	30 days
Oral formulations that contain water	14 days (refrigerated)

*The BUD of the compounded preparation must not exceed the expiration date of any of its ingredients.

COMMON COMPOUNDING EQUIPMENT

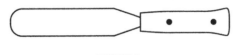

SPATULA

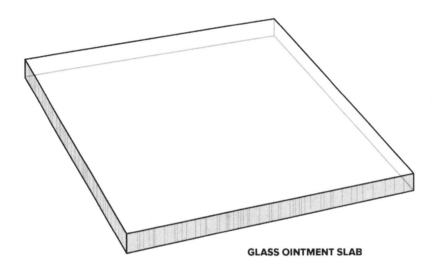

GLASS OINTMENT SLAB

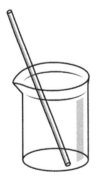

**BEAKER &
GLASS STIRRING ROD**

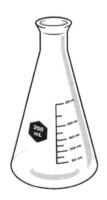

ERLENMEYER FLASK

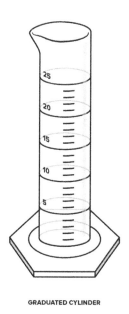

GRADUATED CYLINDER

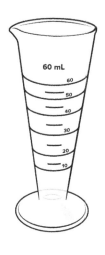

CONICAL GRADUATE

PESTLE ⟶

MORTAR

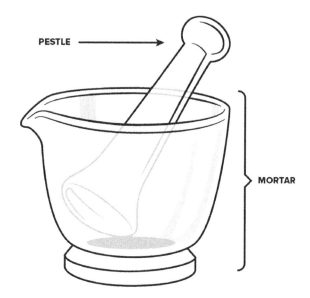

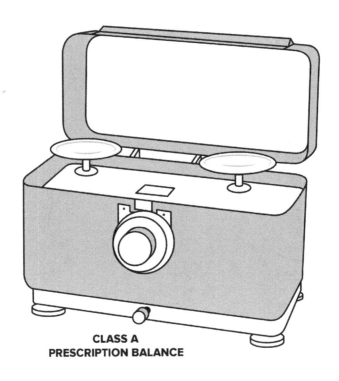

**CLASS A
PRESCRIPTION BALANCE**

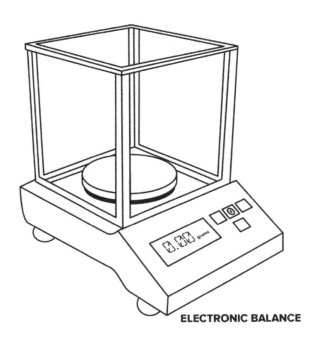

ELECTRONIC BALANCE

Note: A class A prescription balance is the standard, traditional balance used in pharmacies for measuring the weight of ingredients when compounding medications. Most pharmacists these days use an electronic balance, which is easier to use and potentially more accurate.

THE CORRECT METHOD FOR MEASURING LIQUIDS

Look at the image below. If each hash mark represents one milliliter, how many milliliters of gray liquid are contained in the measuring device?

A. 32 mL
B. 31 mL
C. 30 mL
D. 29 mL

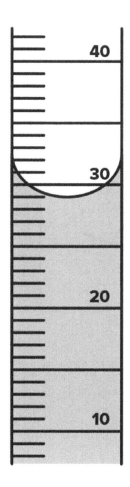

See the following page for an answer and explanation.

ANSWER: D. 29 mL

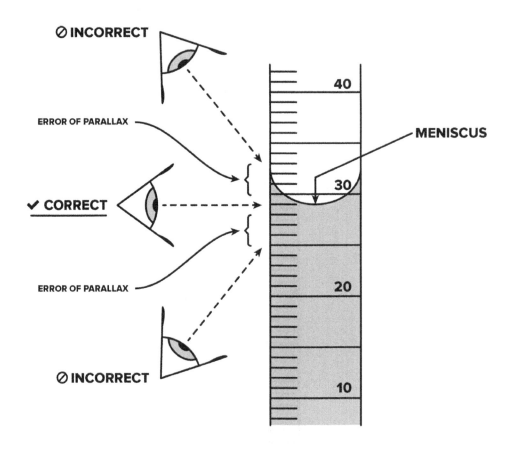

There is only one correct way to measure a liquid using a liquid measuring device, and that is *at the bottom of the meniscus* (the curve at the surface of the liquid) *at eye level*. When measurements are made above or below eye level, the difference between the actual level and the apparent level is called the "error of parallax."

NONSTERILE COMPOUNDING TERMS AND TECHNIQUES

DILUENT
A diluent is an excipient (i.e., an inactive ingredient) that can be added to the preparation to reduce the strength of concentration of the active pharmaceutical ingredient(s).

SPATULATION
The process of mixing two substances (e.g., powders, ointments) on an ointment slab using a spatula to heap the substances together and then flatten them out repeatedly until a homogenous mixture is produced.

TRITURATION
The process of reducing the particle size of a substance, usually by grinding with a mortar and pestle.

LEVIGATION
The process of reducing the particle size of a substance by wetting it with a small amount of insoluble liquid and then triturating or spatulating.

PULVERIZATION BY INTERVENTION
The process of reducing the particle size of a substance by dissolving it in a volatile solvent, then allowing the solvent to evaporate, yielding smaller-sized particles.

ALIQUOT METHOD
Diluting an active pharmaceutical ingredient so a small, otherwise unmeasurable amount can be obtained. This is necessary in some cased because drug doses are often very small (in the microgram to milligram range). Accurately measuring these small doses can be challenging. The standard pharmacy balance is a class A prescription balance, which is sensitive enough to measure 120 mg (or more) within 5% error (or less). To accurately measure smaller quantities with a class A prescription balance, there are two options: #1 attempt to make the measurement with a highly sensitive analytical balance (if possible) or #2 take a larger-than-desired, yet measurable, portion of the drug and dilute it with a known amount of diluent to expand the mass of the substance while decreasing the concentration.

EXAMPLE
ALIQUOT METHOD

If you want to measure 60 mg of a drug using a class A prescription balance, you could take 120 mg (the lowest quantity that can be accurately measured with this type of balance) of the pure (100%) drug powder and mix it with 120 mg of lactose (an inert substance; diluent). Now you have a powder that is 50% drug and 50% lactose. Now you can measure 120 mg of this mixture to obtain 60 mg of the drug. The trick is never to use the balance to measure any quantity less than 120 mg. If you do, you will not stay within the 5% error requirement.

GEOMETRIC DILUTION

Mixing a small amount of one substance with a large amount of another substance by mixing equal portions in several stages to ensure a homogenous mixture is achieved.

EXAMPLE
GEOMETRIC DILUTION

In this example, we need to dilute 200 mg of amlodipine powder with 1,400 mg (a relatively large amount) of lactose powder to form a homogeneous mixture with a total mass of 1,600 mg. To accomplish this using geometric dilution, we will mix the 200 mg of amlodipine with an equal amount (200 mg) of diluent, triturating (or spatulating) until the mixture appears homogeneous. Next, we will add 400 mg of diluent to the 400-mg amlodipine-lactose mixture that was just created in the previous step, triturating (or spatulating) again until the mixture appears homogeneous. Then, as in the previous step, we continue by increasing the amount of lactose added in a stepwise fashion until all of the lactose is added. See the illustration below for visual aid.

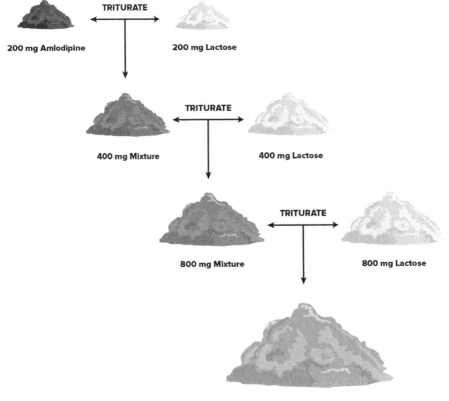

Key Point: If you were to triturate 200 mg of amlodipine with 1,400 mg of lactose all at once, the resultant mixture would likely be uneven (heterogeneous). By slowly adding the diluent in this stepwise fashion (i.e., using geometric dilution), the likelihood of achieving an even (homogeneous) mixture is significantly increased.

PERCENT ERROR AND SENSITIVITY REQUIREMENT

PERCENT ERROR

The difference between the value approximated by a measuring device and the exact actual value. For instance, if the weight of a substance is measured with 5% error, that means that the measurement shown in the measuring device is within +/- 5% of the actual weight of the substance. In pharmacy, the highest acceptable percent error is typically 5% but may be even lower in some cases.

SENSITIVITY REQUIREMENT

The mass needed to move the balance marker by one space (see the illustration below). For a class A prescription balance, the sensitivity requirement is 6 mg.

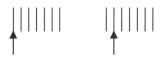

THE RELATIONSHIP BETWEEN SENSITIVITY REQUIREMENT AND PERCENT ERROR

$$\% \text{ Error} = \frac{\text{Sensitivity Requirement}}{\text{Desired Weight}} \times 100\%$$

EXAMPLE #1

Given that the sensitivity requirement of a class A prescription balance is 6 mg, what is the minimum quantity that can be weighed within 5% error?

SOLUTION: This problem can be solved using the above equation. The terms were re-written to reflect the nature of this specific question. **NOTE:** LWQ = least weighable quantity.

$$\text{Maximum Acceptable } \% \text{ Error} = \frac{\text{Sensitivity Requirement}}{\text{LWQ}} \times 100\%$$

$$5\% = \frac{6 \text{ mg}}{\text{LWQ}} \times 100\%$$

Rearrange the equation to solve for LWQ...

$$\text{LWQ} = \frac{6 \text{ mg}}{5\%} \times 100\% = 120 \text{ mg}$$

ANSWER: 120 mg

EXAMPLE #2

What is the percent error if using a class A prescription balance to measure 20 mg of Powder X?

SOLUTION:

$$\% \text{ Error} = \frac{\text{Sensitivity Requirement}}{\text{Desired Weight}} \times 100\% = \frac{6 \text{ mg}}{20 \text{ mg}} \times 100\% = 30\%$$

ANSWER: 30% error

NOTE: 30% error is unacceptable. The highest acceptable level of error is 5% for most preparations.

FOLLOW-UP QUESTION

How could one measure 20 mg of Powder X with a percent error of ≤ 5% using a class A prescription balance? Take 120 mg of the substance (which *can* be measured within 5% error) and use the aliquot method with geometric dilution to create a mixture containing 1 part (120 mg) Powder X and 5 parts (600 mg) diluent. Then, using the class A prescription balance, measure 120 mg of the mixture, which will contain 20 mg of Powder X.

Which of the following pieces of equipment should be used to measure 40 mL of liquid?
A.   10-mL graduated cylinder
B.   50-ml graduated cylinder
C.   20-mL syringe
D.   60-mL syringe

ANSWER: B. 50-mL graduated cylinder

EQUIPMENT SELECTION TIP
USE THE SMALLEST MEASURING DEVICE THAT WILL HOLD THE DESIRED VOLUME

PRACTICE PROBLEMS

1. You want to measure 10 mg of a substance within 1% error without diluting it. The sensitivity requirement of your balance would need to be ___.

2. You are using a class A prescription balance to measure 9 grams of maltose. What percent error will you get with this measurement?

3. You want to measure out 20 mg of hydrocortisone within 5% error using a class A prescription balance. Since the LWQ (least weighable quantity) is 120 mg, you know you will have to perform a geometric dilution to obtain a 20 mg measurement within 5% error. How much diluent powder and hydrocortisone will need to be combined to perform the geometric dilution?

4. After completing the geometric dilution from *practice problem 3* (above), what is the ratio of hydrocortisone to diluent powder?

5. From practice problem 3, what is the percent concentration of hydrocortisone in the resulting powder mixture?

6. From practice problem 3, what is the fraction of hydrocortisone in the resulting powder mixture?

PRACTICE PROBLEM ANSWERS

1. 0.1 mg
2. 0.067%
3. 600 mg of diluent powder & 120 mg of hydrocortisone
4. 1:5 hydrocortisone to diluent powder
5. 16.67%
6. 1/6

MEASUREMENT SYSTEMS

There are three (3) systems of measurement used in pharmacy.

1. The apothecaries' system
2. The avoirdupois system
3. The metric system

The Apothecaries' System

Used in ancient Greece, the apothecaries' system is, for the most part, outdated, but a few older drugs do still have strengths that are expressed in units of grains. Examples include aspirin, ferrous sulfate, Armour Thyroid, nitroglycerin, and phenobarbital. In this system, the grain is the smallest unit of weight, and the minim is the smallest unit of volume.

Weight
1 grain (gr) = 64.8 milligrams
1 scruple (Э) = 20 grains
1 dram (Ʒ) = 3 scruples
1 ounce (Ʒ) = 8 drams
1 pound = 12 ounces

Volume
1 minim (℥) ~ 0.0617 mL
1 fluid dram = 60 minims
1 fluid ounce = 8 fluid drams
1 pint = 16 fluid ounces
1 quart = 2 pints
1 gallon = 4 quarts

The Avoirdupois System

The avoirdupois measurement system is the customary system of weights and measures in the United States. In this system, one (1) pound equals 16 ounces.

Weight
1 grain = 64.8 mg
1 ounce (oz) = 437.5 grains
1 pound lb) = 16 ounces

Volume
1 fluid ounce = 29.57 mL
1 cup = 8 fluid ounces
1 pint = 2 cups
1 quart = 2 pints
1 gallon = 4 quarts

The Metric System

The metric system is the standard measurement system for pharmacy and medicine. As a base-ten system, it is also the simplest measurement system.

Weight
1 milligram (mg) = 1,000 micrograms
1 gram (g) = 1,000 milligrams
1 kilogram (kg) = 1,000 grams

Volume
1 milliliter (mL) = 1 cm^3 (cc)
1 deciliter (dL) = 100 milliliters
1 liter (L) = 1,000 milliliters

ROMAN NUMERALS

ROMAN NUMERALS
I = 1
V = 5
X = 10
L = 50
C = 100
D = 500
M = 1,000

RULES

1) When Roman numerals are repeated, add them together.
    o   Example: III = I + I + I = 3
2) When a smaller Roman numeral is written to the right of a larger Roman numeral, add them together.
    o   Example: VI = V + I = 6
3) When a smaller Roman numeral is written to the left of a larger Roman numeral, subtract it from the larger Roman numeral.
    o   Example IX = X – I = 9
4) Do not use more than three of the same Roman numerals in a sequence.
    o   Example: IIII = 4   IV = 4
5) When rules 2 and 3 conflict, use rule 3.
    o   Example: XIX = 21   XIX = 19

EXAMPLES

Roman numeral XII = 12
Roman numeral XXIV = 24
Roman numeral LIX = 59

PRACTICE PROBLEMS

Convert these numbers to Roman numerals:

1. 120
2. 80
3. 30
4. 3750
5. 1200
6. 473
7. 15
8. 291

Convert these Roman numerals to numbers:

9. CL
10. XC
11. LXV
12. XLVIII
13. MM
14. CCXL
15. CDLXXX
16. CCLVI

PRACTICE PROBLEM ANSWERS

1. CXX
2. LXXX
3. XXX
4. MMMDCCL
5. MCC
6. CDLXXIII
7. XV
8. CCXCI

9. 150
10. 90
11. 65
12. 48
13. 2000
14. 240
15. 480
16. 256

AVERAGES

There are three ways to express an average: Mean, Median, and Mode.

Mean – Add up all the values and divide by the number of values.
> *Example*
> Seven values are given: 1, 4, 6, 3, 9, 8, 3
> Add the seven values: $1 + 4 + 6 + 3 + 9 + 8 + 3 = 34$
> Divide by seven: $34 \div 7 = 4.9$
> Mean = 4.9

Median – Identify the middle value.
> *Example*
> Nine values are given: 11, 3, 10, 5, 4, 5, 5, 8, 7
> Rearrange values into chronological order: 3, 4, 5, 5, 5, 7, 8, 10, 11
> Determine the middle number: 3, 4, 5, 5, 5, 7, 8, 10, 11
> Median = 5

Mode – Identify the value that appears most often in a set of values.
> *Example*
> Eight values are given: 4, 6, 7, 1, 3, 1, 3, 1
> Tally the number of times each value is presented and identify the most commonly presented value:
> 1: III
> 3: II
> 4: I
> 6: I
> 7: I
> Mode = 1

EXAMPLE

A patient measured her blood glucose level daily for one week. Based on her measurements, what was her mean blood glucose for the week?

Monday: 190 mg/dL
Tuesday: 182 mg/dL
Wednesday: 110 mg/dL
Thursday: 90 mg/dL

Friday: 125 mg/dL
Saturday: 130 mg/dL
Sunday: 70 mg/dL

SOLUTION:

$$\frac{(190 + 182 + 110 + 90 + 125 + 130 + 70) \text{ mg/dL}}{7} = 128 \text{ mg/dL}$$

ANSWER: 128 mg/dL

PRACTICE PROBLEMS

1. What is the median in the following set of numbers: 19, 12, 49, 34, 101, 67, 1?

2. What is the mode in the following set of numbers: 4, 2, 1, 4, 5, 2, 4, 3, 2, 1, 2, 4, 2?

3. What is the mean in the following set of numbers: 3, 1, 4, 5, 2, 3, 5, 1, 5, 3, 2, 2, 4?

PRACTICE PROBLEM ANSWERS

1. 34
2. 2
3. 3.1

PERCENT CONCENTRATIONS

Weight/Weight % (w/w) = # of grams of API* per 100 grams of preparation.

    Example

    AndroGel® 1% gel contains 1 g testosterone per 100 grams of gel.

    Practice Problem

    How many milligrams of testosterone are contained in one 5-gram packet of AndroGel® 1% gel?

$$\frac{1\text{ g of testosterone}}{100\text{ g of gel}} \times \frac{5\text{ g of gel}}{1} \times \frac{1{,}000\text{ mg}}{g} = 50\text{ mg of testosterone}$$

Weight/Volume % (w/v) = # of grams of API* per 100 mL of preparation.

    Example

    Clindamycin 1% topical solution contains 1 g clindamycin per 100 mL of solution.

    Practice Problem

    What is the percent concentration (w/v) of a 250-mL solution that contains 35 mg of an active ingredient?

$$\frac{0.035\text{ g}}{250\text{ mL}} = \frac{x}{100\text{ mL}} \quad \therefore \quad x = \frac{0.035\text{ g} \times 100\text{ mL}}{250\text{ mL}} = 0.014\text{ g}$$

$$0.014\text{ g per }100\text{ mL} = 0.014\%\text{ (w/v)}$$

Volume/Volume % (v/v) = # of mL of API* per 100 mL of preparation.

    Example

    Cheratussin® AC contains 3.8% (v/v) alcohol, meaning that there are 3.8-mL of alcohol in every 100-mL of Cheratussin® AC.

    Practice Problem

    What is the percent concentration (v/v) of a 15-mL bottle of a solution that contains 0.75-mL tea tree oil in sterile water?

$$\frac{0.75\text{ mL of API}}{15\text{ mL}} = \frac{x}{100\text{ mL}} \quad \therefore \quad \frac{0.75\text{ mL of API} \times 100\text{ mL}}{15\text{ mL}} = 5\text{ mL}$$

$$5\text{ mL per }100\text{ mL} = 5\%\text{ (v/v)}$$

    Note: API = active pharmaceutical ingredient

When expressing a concentration as a percent, why is it necessary to specify whether the concentration is in terms of w/w, w/v, or v/v?

It is necessary to specify because some substances can only be measured feasibly by weight (solids), while some substances are easier to measure by volume (liquids). Weight and volume are not equal (e.g., 1 mL of alcohol weighs 0.79 grams), except in the case of water (1 mL of water weighs 1 gram). This is because different substances have different densities (see the section titled "Density and Specific Gravity" for more details on density).

PRACTICE PROBLEMS

1. A 6-month-old female is given one-half dropperful of Sodium Fluoride 0.11% (w/v) drops. How many milligrams of Sodium Fluoride did she receive?
Note: 1 dropperful = 1 mL

2. Clobetasol propionate topical solution comes in a 50-mL bottle. If each mL of solution contains 0.5 mg of clobetasol propionate, what is the percent concentration of the solution?

3. Prednisolone 15 mg/5 mL oral solution contains 5% (v/v) alcohol. How many milliliters of alcohol are there in one teaspoonful of solution?

4. Antipyrine and benzocaine otic solution contains 1.4% (w/v) benzocaine and 5.4% (w/v) antipyrine in an anhydrous glycerin base. How many milligrams of each active ingredient are present in one 15-mL bottle?

PRACTICE PROBLEM ANSWERS

1. 0.55 mg Sodium Fluoride
2. 0.05% (w/v)
3. 0.25 mL alcohol
4. 810 mg of antipyrine & 210 mg of benzocaine

RATIOS

THE MAIN PLACES WHERE RATIOS ARE USED IN PHARMACY

#1 In compounding recipes, ratios may be used to quantify the relative amount of each ingredient.
#2 On liquid medication labels, ratios may be used to express the concentration of the active ingredient.

RATIOS IN COMPOUNDING RECIPES

When used in a compounding recipe, ratios describe how many parts of each substance make up the whole. For instance, a 24-ounce cherry pie recipe that calls for a 1:1 ratio of pie dough to cherry filling would be comprised of 12 ounces of pie dough and 12 ounces of cherry filling.

An order for a compounded medication will include the following basic information:
1. The names of each ingredient.
2. The amount or ratio of each ingredient.
3. The amount of final product desired. *

* In some cases, the amount of final product desired may be written by the prescriber as "QS," which comes from the Latin phrase "quantum suffict," meaning "as much as suffices." In this case, you will need to calculate how much to prepare based on the dosing instructions. See the following example.

EXAMPLE #1

What volume of each ingredient will you need to compound the following prescription?

James Smith, D.O.
Simplified Medical Clinic
10001 N. Main St. Suite 100A. Simple City, USA 24680
Telephone# 123-555-1234

Name _George Simpleton_   Age _50_

Address _222 North Main St. Simple City, USA 24680_   Date _1/14/20_

Rx

     1 Part Viscous Lidocaine : 2 Parts Diphenhydramine 12.5 mg/5 mL Elixir

               Dispense QS

       Swish and swallow 3 tsp QID x 14 days

| NR | 1 | 2 | 3 | 4 | 5 | PRN |

James Smith , D.O.

Prescriber must write "Brand Medically Necessary" on the prescription to prohibit generic substitution.

SOLUTION:

Step 1: Since the quantity is written as QS, you must calculate the amount of final product desired. This is easy because you know how much product is being used in one dose (3 teaspoons), you know how many doses the patient will take each day (4 doses/day), and you know how long the patient will be taking the medication (14 days).

$$\frac{15 \text{ mL}}{\text{dose}} \times \frac{4 \text{ doses}}{\text{day}} \times \frac{14 \text{ days}}{1} = 840 \text{ mL}$$

Step 2: Calculate the amount that makes up 1 part of the 3-part mixture by dividing the amount of final product desired by 3 parts.

$$\frac{840 \text{ mL}}{3 \text{ parts}} = 280 \text{ mL/part}$$

Step 3: Now that you know the amount that represents 1 part, calculate the amount of each ingredient that will be needed to compound the prescription.

$$\frac{1 \text{ part of Lidocaine 2\%}}{1} \times \frac{280 \text{ mL}}{\text{part}} = 280 \text{ mL of Lidocaine 2\%}$$

$$\frac{2 \text{ parts Diphenhydramine 12.5/5 mL}}{1} \times \frac{280 \text{ mL}}{\text{part}} = 560 \text{ mL Diphenhydramine 12.5 mg/5 mL}$$

Answer: 280 mL Lidocaine 2% & 560 mL diphenhydramine 12.5 mg/5 mL

Ratios Used to Express the Concentration of a Medication

When used to express a concentration, a ratio describes how many parts of the active ingredient are present in a certain number of parts of the total formulation. For example, epinephrine 1:10,000 solution contains 1 part epinephrine in 10,000 parts of solution. The conversion factors below are for your reference.

CONVERSION FACTORS FOR CONCENTRATIONS EXPRESSED BY A RATIO
1:1 = 1 gram per mL = 1 g/mL
1:1,000 = 1×10^{-3} grams per mL = 1 mg/mL
1:1,000,000 = 1×10^{-6} grams per mL = 1 mcg/mL

EXAMPLE #2

How many milligrams of epinephrine are there in 2 milliliters of Epinephrine 1:1,000,000 solution?

SOLUTION:
Step 1: Convert the ratio into a value with metric units using the conversion factor above.

According to conversion factor above, 1:1,000,000 = 1 mcg/mL

Step 2: Apply the following equation **or** use the unit conversion/proportion approach.

$$\frac{Weight_1}{Volume_1} = \frac{Weight_2}{Volume_2}$$

Insert the given information into the equation.
Weight $_1$ = 1 mcg
Volume $_1$ = 1 mL
Weight $_2$ = ?
Volume $_2$ = 2 mL

$$\frac{1 \ mcg}{1 \ mL} = \frac{Weight_2}{2 \ mL}$$

Step 3: Get the unknown value (Weight$_2$) alone.

$$Weight_2 = \frac{1 \ mcg \ x \ 2 \ mL}{1 \ mL} = 2 \ mcg$$

Answer: 2 mcg

PRACTICE PROBLEMS

1. The package for EpiPen Jr 2-Pak® comes with 2 Auto-Injectors, each one containing 0.3 mL of a 1:2000 epinephrine solution. How many milligrams of epinephrine are in one EpiPen Jr 2-Pak®?

2. What is the ratio strength of a 20-mL solution that contains 200 mcg of a drug?

3. What is the ratio strength of a solution that contains 1 mg of drug per mL of solution?

4. How many milliliters of a 1:200 stock solution of Lidocaine would be required to compound a prescription for 50 mL of 0.25% Lidocaine solution?

5. If you have 1 gallon of a 1:40 solution of Drug XYZ, how many Liters of 1:1,000 solution of Drug XYZ can you compound?

PRACTICE PROBLEM ANSWERS

1. 0.3 mg (0.15 mg of epinephrine per Auto-Injector, and there are two Auto-Injectors in one EpiPen Jr 2-Pak®)
2. 1:10,000
3. 1:1,000
4. 25 mL
5. 94.6 L

ALLIGATION ALTERNATE

Alligation is a great way to solve certain compounding math problems. Use alligation when you are given two products with different concentrations of the same drug, and you need a concentration that falls somewhere in the between (or when you have a higher concentration than what is desired, and you want to dilute it with an inert substance like water or petrolatum). Start by drawing an X with a hollow center.

In every alligation problem, you will have to compound a prescription for a certain concentration using two products. One product will have a higher-than-desired concentration, and the other product will have a lower-than-desired concentration. For example, let's say we have a 1% cream of Product B and a 10% cream of Product B, and we want to make a cream that contains 3% Product B. Write the value for the high concentration product at the top left, and write the value for the low concentration product at the bottom left.

Next, write the value of the desired concentration in the center.

Then calculate the difference between the numbers on the left side of the X and the number at the center. Write the answer, following the diagonal line, at the opposite corner of the X.

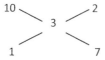

The numbers on the right side of the X indicate the proportion of each ingredient needed to compound a formulation of the desired concentration.

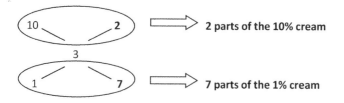

At this point, you would have all the information needed to solve the problem. Let's say the prescription called for 60 grams of 3% Product B cream. Based on the results of the alligation, you know that the cream would be made up of nine equal parts (2 parts of 10% cream and 7 parts of 1% cream). Divide 60 grams into nine equal parts (60 g ÷ 9 parts = 6.67 g/part). You would need 13.3 g (6.67 g/part x 2 parts = 13.3 g) of 10% cream and 46.7 g (6.67 g/part x 7 parts = 46.7 g) of 1% cream to compound 60 g of 3 % Product B cream. Now, practice as many of these as you can!

EXAMPLE #1

You need 30 g of Triamcinolone 0.05% ointment, but all you have in stock is Triamcinolone 0.025% and 0.1% ointment. How much of each ingredient will you need in order to compound this prescription?

SOLUTION:

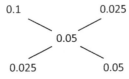

$$0.025 : 0.05 = 1 : 2$$

1 part of 0.1% triamcinolone : 2 parts of 0.025% triamcinolone

$$\frac{30 \text{ g}}{3 \text{ parts}} \times \frac{1 \text{ part of 0.1\% triamcinolone}}{1} = 10 \text{ g of 0.1\% triamcinolone}$$

$$\frac{30 \text{ g}}{3 \text{ parts}} \times \frac{2 \text{ parts of 0.025\% triamcinolone}}{1} = 20 \text{ g of 0.025\% triamcinolone}$$

ANSWER: 10 g of 0.1% and 20 g of 0.025% triamcinolone ointment

---

EXAMPLE #2

You have 800 mL of 70% alcohol solution. How much water will you need to add to make a 10% alcohol solution? NOTE: Assume the water contains 0% alcohol

SOLUTION:

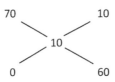

10 parts = 800 mL ∴ 1 part = 80 mL

$$60 \text{ parts} \times \frac{80 \text{ mL}}{\text{part}} = 4{,}800 \text{ mL}$$

ANSWER: 4,800 mL of water

EXAMPLE #3

How many grams of pure Sodium Chloride must be added to 10 mL of normal saline solution to create a 3% NaCl solution? NOTE: Pure NaCl is 100% NaCl

SOLUTION:

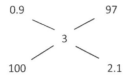

$$97 \text{ parts of } 0.9\% \text{ NaCl} = 10 \text{ mL} \therefore 1 \text{ part} = \frac{10 \text{ mL}}{97} = 0.103 \text{ mL}$$

$$2.1 \text{ parts x } \frac{0.103 \text{ mL}}{\text{part}} = 0.22 \text{ mL} \sim 0.22 \text{ g}$$

ANSWER: 0.22 g of pure NaCl

EXAMPLE #4

You need to compound an IV solution of 2.5 mg/mL Vancomycin in D5W using a vial that contains 1 gram of Vancomycin in 20 mL. How much D5W will be needed?

SOLUTION:
<u>Step 1</u>: Convert the concentrations to percentages.

Note: A one-percent solution contains one gram per one hundred milliliters (1% = 1 g/100 mL). Knowing this, you can convert the given units to a percentage by calculating the number of grams in 100 mL.

Desired Concentration (To Be Compounded)

$$\frac{2.5 \text{ mg}}{\text{mL}} \text{ x } \frac{1 \text{ g}}{1,000 \text{ mg}} \text{ x } 100 \text{ mL} = 0.25 \text{ g}$$

If 100 mL of the solution contains 0.25 g of Vancomycin, then the percent concentration would be 0.25%.

Given Concentration (In Vial)

$$\frac{1 \text{ g}}{20 \text{ mL}} \text{ x } 5 = \frac{5 \text{ g}}{100 \text{ mL}} = 5\%$$

To summarize, we are given a 5% Vancomycin solution, and we want to create a 0.25% Vancomycin solution using D5W (contains 0% Vancomycin).

Step 2: Alligation math.

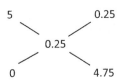

0.25 parts of 5% Vancomycin : 4.75 parts of D5W

In other words (if you multiply each part by a factor of 4), the compound must be made up of 1 part of 5% Vancomycin and 19 parts D5W.

We know we are using 20 mL of the 5% Vancomycin solution, so:

1 part = 20 mL ∴ 19 parts = 19 x 20 mL = 380 mL

ANSWER: 380 mL of D5W

PRACTICE PROBLEMS

1. How much of each ingredient will be needed to make 50 mL of 1% KCl solution from 3% KCl solution and water?

2. How many Liters of 3% H_2O_2 and 6% H_2O_2 will you need to mix to make 2 Liters of 4.5% H_2O_2?

3. You need to dilute a 5% Lidocaine cream to compound 45 grams of 4% Lidocaine cream using a cream base. How much 5% Lidocaine cream will be needed to compound this prescription?

4. How many grams of 1% Hydrocortisone cream will need to be mixed with 100% Hydrocortisone powder to make 2 ounces of 2.5% Hydrocortisone cream? **NOTE:** 1 ounce = 28.35 grams

---

PRACTICE PROBLEM ANSWERS

1. 16.7 mL of 3% KCl solution; 33.3 mL of water
2. 1 Liter of 3% H_2O_2 & 1 Liter of 6% H_2O_2
3. 36 grams of 5% Lidocaine cream
4. 55.8 grams of 1% Hydrocortisone cream

PROPORTIONS AND UNIT CONVERSION

Most of the math you will face on the PTCB exam involves proportions. The following is an example of a proportion:

$$\frac{a}{b} = \frac{c}{d}$$

When you get a proportion problem, you must first cross multiply. For example:

$$\frac{a}{b} = \frac{c}{d} \quad \therefore \quad a \times d = b \times c$$

Then isolate the unknown. For instance:

$$a = \frac{b \times c}{d} \quad \text{or} \quad b = \frac{a \times d}{c} \quad \text{or} \quad c = \frac{a \times d}{b} \quad \text{or} \quad d = \frac{b \times c}{a}$$

Here is an example of a real-life problem that involves proportions:
A car travels at a speed of 60 miles per hour. How many miles does the car travel in 2.5 hours?

$$\frac{60 \text{ miles}}{1 \text{ hour}} = \frac{? \text{ miles}}{2.5 \text{ hours}} \quad \therefore \quad ? \text{ miles} = \frac{60 \text{ miles} \times 2.5 \text{ hours}}{1 \text{ hour}} = 150 \text{ miles}$$

Be sure that the units match on each side of the proportion. For instance, let's say the question was: how many miles were traveled in 150 <u>minutes</u>?

To solve this problem, you would first need to convert the units from minutes to hours like this:

$$150 \text{ minutes} \times \frac{1 \text{ hour}}{60 \text{ minutes}} = 2.5 \text{ hours}$$

These units cancel out.

Many pharmacy calculations are quickly solved using the same approach. For instance, let's say you dispense 50 tablets to a patient that takes 2 tablets per day. How many days will the bottle of 50 tablets last?

$$50 \text{ tablets} \times \frac{\text{day}}{2 \text{ tablets}} = 25 \text{ days}$$

The term 1 hour/60 minutes is a "conversion factor." When we multiplied 150 minutes by 1hour/60 minutes, we essentially multiplied the value 150 minutes by a factor of 1. Why? Because this calculation did not increase or decrease the amount of time the car was traveling, it just changed the units used to express the amount of time traveled (150 minutes and 2.5 hours are the same). You will use conversion factors frequently when solving pharmacy math problems. For instance, one conversion factor commonly used in pharmacy is 5 milliliters/teaspoonful (can also be expressed as 1 teaspoonful/5 milliliters). You need to memorize this conversion factor and a few others (see the list of **Must-Know Conversion Factors** in the section titled "The Secret to Solving Nearly Any Pharmacy Math Problem").

THE SECRET TO SOLVING NEARLY ANY PHARMACY MATH PROBLEM

The secret is simple – in fact, we have already begun to reveal the secret – it is simply unit conversion. Many textbooks try to teach a more complex version of this concept that is unnecessarily difficult. The approach I am about to teach you is the same one that I successfully use to solve nearly *all* of the problems I encounter in my everyday work. The best advice to mastering this approach is to work through a lot of examples and practice problems (plenty of which you will find on the following pages). You will see this problem-solving approach applied throughout this study guide. First, memorize the **Must-Know Conversion Factors** (listed below) and the **Common Pharmacy Math Equations** (listed in Appendix A on page 239). Then, move on to the next page and begin solving problems! Below is the general equation you will use:

(# in Given Units) x (Conversion Factor*) = # in Desired Units

*Conversion Factor = Desired Units/Given Units

MUST-KNOW CONVERSION FACTORS

VOLUME
1 cubic centimeter (cc) = 1 milliliter (mL)
1 Liter (L) = 1,000 mL
1 teaspoon (tsp) = 5 mL
1 tablespoon (tbsp) = 3 tsp = 15 mL
1 fluid ounce (volume) = 29.57 mL*
Most pharmacists round up to 30 mL
1 Cup = 8 fluid ounces (fl oz)
1 Pint = 2 cups
1 Quart = 2 pints
1 Gallon = 4 quarts

WEIGHT
1 milligram (mg) = 1,000 micrograms
1 gram (g) = 1,000 mg
1 kilogram (kg) = 1,000 g
1 kg = 2.2 pounds (lb)
1 ounce (oz) = 28.35 g
1 lb = 454 g
1 grain (gr) = 64.8 mg

HEIGHT
1 inch (in) = 2.54 centimeters (cm)

Solving pharmacy math problems is all about combining given variables with known values (such as those shown above) to calculate the answer.

1) Identify the given variables:
   The information provided in the problem/question.
2) Remember the known values:
   The **Must-Know Conversion Factors** and the **Common Pharmacy Math Equations**.
3) Calculate the answer:
   Multiply, divide, and/or apply the relevant equation to determine the answer.

EXAMPLE #1

A 5-year-old child has a cardiac arrhythmia. To treat the arrhythmia, the doctor prescribes propranolol at the daily dose of 0.5 mg/kg. If we determine that the child weighs 55 pounds, how many milligrams of propranolol should the child receive each day?

Given variables (provided by the question above):
Age = 5 years old
Dose = 0.5 mg/kg
Weight = 55 lb

Known values (memorized from the previous page):
Must-Know Conversion Factors
Common Pharmacy Math Equations

Calculate the answer:
Using what you are given and what you know, determine how many milligrams of the medication the patient should receive each day. Everything you need to solve the problem comes from what you are given and/or what you know from memorizing the values on the previous page. All you have to do is take this information and make the units change and/or cancel out until you get the desired units.

The dose is already given in the question as 0.5 mg/kg. Now, just find a way to get the kilogram units to cancel out, and then you will have the dose in milligrams.

$$\frac{0.5 \text{ mg}}{kg} \times ? \times ?... = ? \text{ mg}$$

What factor(s) must you multiply by to get an answer in milligrams?

Now is the time to look back at "what you are given" and "what you know" to identify the factors you can use to cancel out the kilogram units and obtain your answer in milligrams.

Given variables:
~~Age = 5 years old~~ (age is irrelevant because the dose is based on weight)

Dose = 0.5 mg/kg

Weight = 55 lb

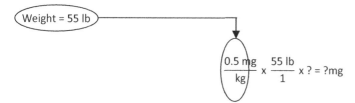

The child's weight is given in the question. If only the weight was in units of kilograms, then you would be able to solve the problem.

Known values:

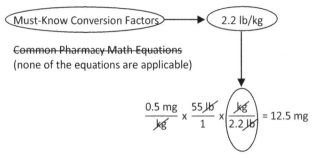

CORRECT ANSWER: 12.5 mg

The key to solving this problem was taking what you were given, combining it with what you know, and then figuring out which pieces of information were relevant for obtaining an answer in the desired units.

EXAMPLE #2

How many fluid ounces (℥) are in 118 mL (please answer in Roman numerals)?

SOLUTION:

> Think of the dividing line as the word "per"

$$\text{\# in Desired Units} = 118 \text{ mL} \times \frac{1 \text{ fluid ounce}}{29.57 \text{ mL}} = 4 \text{ fluid ounces}$$

NOTE: notice how the mL units cancel out.

ANSWER: IV ℥ (4 fluid ounces)

***There are 29.57 milliliters **per** fluid ounce (29.57 mL/fluid ounce). This can be written as "29.57 mL/1 fluid ounce" **or** "1 fluid ounce/29.57 mL." Since 1 fluid ounce is *equal* to 29.57 mL, then 29.57 mL ÷ 1 fluid ounce = 1.

Multiplying a value by the factor "29.57 mL/1 fluid ounce" is like multiplying it by 1. The actual value doesn't change, but the units do change. This is true when you multiply any number by a conversion factor.

Since multiplying by the factor "29.57 mL/1 fluid ounce" is mathematically the same as multiplying by 1, multiplying the reciprocal "1 fluid ounce/29.57 mL" is also like multiplying by 1. How do you know which way to orient the conversion factor? You have to decide which units you want on top (the numerator), and which units you want on the bottom (the denominator) based on what units you are trying to obtain. The units you are trying to obtain should go in the numerator and the units you are trying to eliminate should go in the denominator. See below for an example of what happens when you orient the conversion factor **incorrectly**:

$$118 \text{ mL} \times \frac{29.57 \text{ mL}}{1 \text{ fluid ounce}} = 3{,}489 \text{ mL}^2/\text{fluid ounce}$$

...clearly, this did not lead to an answer with the desired units.

EXAMPLE #3

How many kilograms (kg) does a 77 lb patient weigh?

SOLUTION:

$$\text{\# in Desired Units} = 77 \text{ lb} \times \frac{\text{kg}}{2.2 \text{ lb}} = 35 \text{ kg}$$

ANSWER: 35 kg

EXAMPLE #4

How many milliliters are in 16 ounces?

SOLUTION:

$$\text{\# in Desired Units} = 16 \text{ ounces} \times \frac{29.57 \text{ mL}}{\text{ounce}} = 473 \text{ mL}$$

NOTE: Milliliters (mL) are the "Desired Units" because the question asks for an answer in milliliters. Likewise, the # in Given Units is 16 ounces, as that is the value we are given. Since we know the conversion factor (29.57 mL per ounce), we have all the information needed to solve the problem.

ANSWER: 473 mL

EXAMPLE #5

A patient drops off a prescription for 30 tablets of 5-grain ferrous sulfate. You only have four iron products stocked in the pharmacy. Which of the four products should you dispense?

A. Fergon® (Ferrous gluconate 250 mg)
B. Ferro-Sequels® (Ferrous fumarate 150 mg)
C. Feosol® (Ferrous sulfate 325 mg)
D. SlowFe® (Ferrous sulfate 225 mg)

SOLUTION:

$$\text{\# in Desired Units} = \frac{5 \text{ grains}}{1} \times \frac{64.8 \text{ mg}}{\text{grain}} = 324 \text{ mg}$$

ANSWER: C. Feosol® (Ferrous sulfate 325 mg)

Note: The answer we calculated was 1 mg lower than the answer we selected. Why is this alright? Many times, the value of 1 grain is rounded up to 65 mg. If you were to use 1 grain = 65 mg as the conversion factor (rather than 1 grain = 64.8 mg), your answer would be 325 mg. The difference is not significant, so either strength is acceptable.

EXAMPLE #6

You receive a prescription order for Nitrostat® sublingual tablets 1/200 grain. Nitrostat® sublingual tablets are available in 3 strengths. Which strength should you dispense?

A. 0.3 mg
B. 0.4 mg
C. 0.6 mg

SOLUTION:

$$\text{\# in Desired Units} = \frac{1 \text{ grain}}{200} \times \frac{64.8 \text{ mg}}{\text{grain}} = 0.3 \text{ mg}$$

ANSWER: A. 0.3 mg

EXAMPLE #7

An order comes to the pharmacy for levothyroxine 0.125 mg IV injection. Using a levothyroxine 40 mcg/mL solution, how many milliliters should you dispense?

A. 0.0031 mL
B. 3.1 mL
C. 0.31 mL
D. 3.1 μL

SOLUTION:

$$\text{\# in Desired Units} = \frac{0.125 \text{ mg}}{1} \times \frac{1,000 \text{ mcg}}{\text{mg}} \times \frac{\text{mL}}{40 \text{ mcg}} = 3.1 \text{ mL}$$

ANSWER: B. 3.1 mL

EXAMPLE #8

A patient weighs 100.1 kg. What is the patient's weight in pounds?

SOLUTION:

$$\text{\# in Desired Units} = \frac{100.1 \text{ kg}}{1} \times \frac{2.2 \text{ lb}}{\text{kg}} = 220 \text{ lb}$$

ANSWER: 220 lb

EXAMPLE #9

The Glucagon Emergency Kit for Low Blood Sugar, manufactured by Lilly, comes with a vial containing 1 mg of glucagon and 49 mg of lactose. Assuming Lilly has all the glucagon it needs, how many vials can they prepare using only one pound of lactose?

SOLUTION:

$$\frac{1 \text{ lb of lactose}}{1} \times \frac{16 \text{ ounces}}{\text{pound}} \times \frac{28.35 \text{ g}}{\text{ounce}} \times \frac{1,000 \text{ mg}}{\text{g}} = 453,600 \text{ mg of lactose}$$

$$\frac{453,600 \text{ mg of lactose}}{1} \times \frac{\text{vial}}{49 \text{ mg of lactose}} = 9,257 \text{ vials}$$

ANSWER: 9,257 vials

SOMETIMES THE CONVERSION FACTOR IS GIVEN IN THE QUESTION
SEE BELOW FOR EXAMPLE

EXAMPLE #10

What is the days' supply of a bottle of 90 tablets of levothyroxine 112 mcg if the instructions are to take one tablet by mouth every day, except take one-half tablet on Sundays?

SOLUTION:

$$\frac{90 \text{ tablets}}{1} \times \frac{7 \text{ days}}{6.5 \text{ tablets}} = 96.9 \text{ days} \therefore 97 \text{ days}$$

Note: The conversion factor here was 6.5 tablets/7 days.

ANSWER: 97 days

EXAMPLE #11

Given a solution that contains 100 mg of drug per 5 mL, how many milliliters would be required to obtain a dose of 650 mg?

SOLUTION:

$$\frac{650 \text{ mg}}{1} \times \frac{5 \text{ mL}}{100 \text{ mg}} = 32.5 \text{ mL}$$

ANSWER: 32.5 mL

EXAMPLE #12

Sometimes, you will need to do a series of conversions to reach the answer you need. Take this problem, for example: How many 75 mcg tablets can be made from six pounds of a drug?

Solution:

$$\frac{6 \text{ pounds}}{1} \times \frac{16 \text{ ounces}}{lb} \times \frac{28.35 \text{ g}}{ounce} \times \frac{1,000,000 \text{ mcg}}{g} \times \frac{tablet}{75 \text{ mcg}} = 36,288,000 \text{ tablets}$$

Answer: 36,288,000 tablets

PRACTICE PROBLEMS

1. How many fluid ounces are in a jug containing 3,785 mL of polyethylene glycol with electrolytes?

2. After reconstitution, how many teaspoons are in three 100-mL bottles of Amoxicillin 250 mg/5 mL oral suspension? Express your answer in Roman numerals.

3. Approximately how many tablespoons are in a 4 oz bottle of cough syrup?

4. How many scruples of aspirin are in sixteen 5 grain tablets of Ecotrin®?

5. If a patient is 6 feet tall, how tall would the patient be in centimeters?

6. You have 7 pounds of triamcinolone 0.1% ointment. How many kilograms do you have?

7. How many tablespoons are in a 150-mL bottle of an antibiotic suspension?

8. How many milliliters of a 200 mg/mL solution of testosterone cypionate should be injected intramuscularly if the patient needs to receive 75 mg per injection?

9. How many milliliters are needed to provide one 300 mg dose of amoxicillin using a 250 mg/5 mL amoxicillin suspension?

10. If a patient applies 4 g of Voltaren® 1% Gel (10 mg diclofenac/1 g gel) to her knee every day, then how many milligrams of diclofenac are being applied daily?

11. A physician wrote a prescription for testosterone cypionate 200 mg/mL solution with the instructions to inject 0.75 mL intramuscularly once every two weeks. How many grams of the drug will the patient inject over the course of one year?

PRACTICE PROBLEM ANSWERS

1.   128 fluid ounces
2.   LX teaspoons
3.   8 tablespoons
4.   4 scruples
5.   183 centimeters
6.   3.18 kilograms
7.   10 tablespoons
8.   0.375 milliliters
9.   6 mL
10. 40 mg
11. 3.9 g

MILLIEQUIVALENTS

Most units of measure can be converted simply by multiplying by the appropriate conversion factor, but milliequivalents (mEq) are the exception to the rule. Milligrams are similar to milliequivalents, but with one simple distinction - milligrams are a measure of mass, whereas milliequivalents are a measure of the concentration of ions. To convert between milligrams (mg) and mEq, use the following equations:

CONVERT FROM mg TO mEq

$$\frac{mg \times Valence}{Molecular\ Weight} = ?\ mEq$$

CONVERT FROM mEq TO mg

$$\frac{mEq \times Molecular\ Weight}{Valence} = ?\ mg$$

Molecular weight is determined by adding the atomic mass of each element in a molecule. You can find atomic mass values in the periodic table. Valence values can be determined from their location in the periodic table, but we created the following chart to summarize the molecular weight and valence values for the most common electrolytes seen in pharmacy practice:

ELECTROLYTE	VALENCE	MOLECULAR WEIGHT
Calcium (Ca^{2+})	2	40
Ferrous (Fe^{2+})	2	56
Ferric (Fe^{3+})	3	56
Lithium (Li^+)	1	7
Magnesium (Mg^{2+})	2	24
Potassium (K^+)	1	39
Sodium (Na^+)	1	23
Carbonate (CO_3^{2-})	2	60
Chloride (Cl^-)	1	35.5
Sulfate (SO_4^{2-})	2	96

EXAMPLE #1

How many milligrams of potassium chloride are in one 20 mEq tablet of potassium chloride (K-Dur®)?

A. 710 mg
B. 780 mg
C. 1,490 mg
D. 1,560 mg

SOLUTION:

$$\frac{mEq \times Molecular\ Weight}{Valence} = ?\ mg$$

$$\frac{20\ mEq \times (39 + 35.5)}{1} = 1,490\ mg$$

ANSWER: C. 1,490 mg

EXAMPLE #2

How many milliequivalents are in 3.54 grams of sodium?

A. 1.54 mEq
B. 3.08 mEq
C. 154 mEq
D. 308 mEq

SOLUTION:

$$\frac{\text{mg x Valence}}{\text{Molecular Weight}} = ? \text{ mEq}$$

$$\frac{3,540 \text{ mg x 1}}{23} = 154 \text{ mEq}$$

ANSWER: C. 154 mEq

DAYS' SUPPLY CALCULATIONS

When insurance companies are billed for prescriptions, the pharmacy technician and pharmacist are responsible for calculating the days' supply being dispensed. If you bill an insurance company for a days' supply less than that actually dispensed (e.g., dispense a 30-day supply of medication and bill the insurance as though it were a 10-day supply) the insurance company can issue a "charge-back" during an audit (i.e. the pharmacy would have to pay the insurance company back; may also be referred to as "recoupment" by insurance companies). The most commonly prescribed medications are available from the manufacturer in the form of tablets or capsules ("solid oral dosage forms"). In these cases, determining the days' supply is a simple one-step calculation.

EXAMPLE #1

What is the days' supply for a prescription of 30 tablets of Drug X with the instructions to take one tablet by mouth once daily?

$$\frac{30 \text{ tablets}}{1} \times \frac{\text{day}}{1 \text{ tablet}} = 30 \text{ days}$$

EXAMPLE #2

What is the days' supply for a prescription of 60 tablets of Drug AB9012 with the instructions to take one tablet three times daily as needed for pain?

$$\frac{60 \text{ tablets}}{1} \times \frac{\text{day}}{3 \text{ tablets}} = 20 \text{ days}$$

Note: When the instructions include the term "as needed," assume the patient will use the maximum amount when calculating the days' supply.

Calculating the days' supply of a non-solid dosage form (e.g., oral liquids, eye drops, ear drops, nasal sprays, and inhalers) can be more challenging. Study the example problems on the next two pages, then practice these calculations yourself until you master them!

USE THE INFORMATION BELOW TO COMPLETE THE PROBLEMS IN THIS SECTION

ProAir®, Proventil®, and Ventolin® each contain 120 puffs/inhaler
Astepro® nasal spray contains 200 sprays/bottle
Flonase® nasal spray contains 120 sprays/bottle
Xalatan® eye drops contain 2.5 mL/bottle

EXAMPLE #3

How many days will a 4-ounce bottle of cetirizine 5 mg/5 mL solution last if the instructions are to take one-half teaspoonful QHS? NOTE: Read the question carefully!

$$\frac{120 \text{ mL}}{\text{bottle}} \times \frac{\text{tsp}}{5 \text{ mL}} \times \frac{\text{day}}{0.5 \text{ tsp}} = 48 \text{ days/bottle}$$

EXAMPLE #4

What would the days' supply be on a prescription for Flonase® nasal spray if the instructions are 1 spray in each nostril QD?

$$\frac{120 \text{ sprays}}{\text{bottle}} \times \frac{\text{day}}{2 \text{ sprays}} = 60 \text{ days/bottle}$$

EXAMPLE #5

Try it yourself: Calculate the days' supply of 1 bottle of Astepro® if the instructions say to instill 1 spray into each nostril BID.

Answer: 50-day supply

EXAMPLE #6

A prescription is written for 3 Ventolin® HFA Inhalers with the instructions to inhale 2 puffs PO Q4-6H PRN wheezing. Each inhaler contains enough medication for 200 puffs. What would the days' supply of this prescription be?

$$\frac{3 \text{ inhalers}}{1} \times \frac{200 \text{ puffs}}{\text{inhaler}} \times \frac{\text{day}}{12 \text{ puffs}} = 50 \text{ days}$$

TEST YOUR KNOWLEDGE

How many drops are in one milliliter (1 mL)?

15–20 drops

EXAMPLE #7

What is the days' supply for a 7.5 mL bottle of Ciprodex® Otic Solution with the instructions: ii gtts AS QID until gone?

    A.   7 days
    B.   10 days
    C.   12 days
    D.   19 days
    E.   25 days

SOLUTION:
<u>Step 1</u>: Interpret the sig.

"ii gtts AS QID until gone"
        = instill two drops into the left ear four times daily until gone.

<u>Step 2</u>: Since the question does not specify how many drops are in one milliliter, calculate the days' supply based on the conversion factor of 20 drops/mL.

$$\frac{7.5 \text{ mL}}{1} \times \frac{20 \text{ drops}}{\text{mL}} \times \frac{\text{day}}{8 \text{ drops}} = 18.75 \text{ days} \therefore 19 \text{ days}$$

ANSWER: D. 19 days

You are dispensing a 5-mL bottle of ciprofloxacin 0.3% ophthalmic solution with instructions to instill two drops into each eye three times daily until gone. What is the days' supply of this prescription (assume 20 drops/mL)?

$$\frac{5 \text{ mL}}{1} \times \frac{20 \text{ drops}}{\text{mL}} \times \frac{\text{day}}{12 \text{ drops}} = 8 \text{ days}$$

THE RULE OF HAND

One (1) gram of topical medication is roughly enough to cover one side (palm and fingers) of four flat hands. Use the Rule of Hand when calculating the days' supply of topical medications.

PRACTICE PROBLEMS

1. What is the days' supply for a 15-gram tube of acne medication with instructions to apply to the entire face nightly? **NOTE:** The area of the face is roughly equal to the area of two flat hands.

2. You are dispensing two Ventolin® HFA inhalers with instructions for the patient to inhale one to two puffs by mouth every four to six hours as needed for shortness of breath. What will the days' supply be for this prescription?

3. What is the days' supply for a quantity of 60 venlafaxine ER 37.5 mg capsules with the following instructions: i PO QD x 7 days, then i PO BID x 7 days, then ii QAM and i QPM thereafter?

4. What is the days' supply for a 120-mL bottle of Tussionex® suspension with the following instructions: take i tsp PO up to TID PRN for cough?

5. You dispense a prescription for methotrexate 2.5 mg tablets with instructions to take three tablets by mouth weekly. What is the days' supply for 30 tablets?

6. NovoLog® FlexPen is available in a package that contains five pens. Each pen contains three milliliters of NovoLog® insulin. If a patient uses 11 units SQ every morning and 9 units SQ every evening with a meal, what is the days' supply for a single package that contains five pens? **Note:** The concentration of NovoLog® insulin is 100 units per milliliter.

7. Antipyrine-benzocaine otic solution comes in a 15-mL bottle. What is the days' supply if the instructions are as follows: instill 2-4 gtts AU up to QID PRN? **NOTE:** Assume there are 20 drops per mL.

PRACTICE PROBLEM ANSWERS

1. 30 days
2. 33 days
3. 27 days
4. 8 days
5. 70 days
6. 75 days
7. 9 days

THE "STEROID TAPER"

The human body naturally produces steroid hormones. Taking medicinal steroids leads to a reduction in the body's internal production of steroids. At high doses, the use of medicinal steroids can shut down steroid hormone production within the body entirely. For this reason, when discontinuing high doses of steroids, it is necessary to decrease the dose gradually over time (as opposed to abruptly stopping the medication) to give the body time to turn steroid production back on. This process of gradual reduction is called a taper.

When doctors prescribe short courses of a high-dose steroid, they will often use a dose pack. An example of a steroid dose pack is the prednisone 10 mg 6-day dose pack, where the patient takes 6 tablets the first day and decreases by one tablet daily until finished (6, 5, 4, 3, 2, 1, stop). With dose packs, the manufacturer includes the instructions directly on the packaging. This makes it more convenient for the patient and the prescriber.

It should be noted that steroid tapers can be accomplished without the use of a dose pack. For instance, a prescriber could issue a prescription for prednisone with instructions to take 30 mg daily for 3 days, 20 mg daily for 3 days, 10 mg daily for 3 days, 5 mg daily for 3 days, and then stop.

Note: The term "taper" can also be used to describe gradually increasing the dose of a medication (also known as "titrating" the dose). Starting at a low dose and increasing it slowly up to the optimal therapeutic dose allows the body to gradually build a tolerance to the drug, thus reducing the incidence of side effects. For example, gabapentin is often initiated at a low dose and then gradually increased to a more effective dose in an attempt to avoid the side effect of drowsiness. Another example is metformin, which is usually dosed in a similar fashion to avoid side effects such as upset stomach and diarrhea.

When dealing with tapers, days' supply calculations can be more challenging. Remember, when an insurance company is improperly billed for a prescription, they can recoup previously paid money in an audit; in other words, the pharmacy must pay them back. For instance, if an insurance company audits your pharmacy and finds that a prescription was dispensed for a 90-day supply, but you billed them as though the prescription were only a 30-day supply, the insurance company can say that the claim was not submitted correctly and demand that the pharmacy pay them back.

Useful Fact: Prednisone dose packs come in two sizes: a 48-tablet 6-day dose pack <u>or</u> a 21-tablet 12-day dose pack.

While we are on the topic, let's talk about the term "dosepak." Some people use the terms "dosepak" and "dose pack" interchangeably. Truth be told, "dosepak" is not a real word; rather, it is a portion of one of Pfizer's brand name drugs, the Medrol® Dosepak™. The name is similar to one of Pfizer's other inventions, the Z-pak®. The names ending in "pak" belong to Pfizer. All other dose packs (such as prednisone dose packs, generic methylprednisolone dose packs, and generic azithromycin dose packs) are just called "dose packs."

DENSITY AND SPECIFIC GRAVITY

Density = mass (grams) per unit volume (milliliters).

$$\text{Density} = \frac{\text{Mass (grams)}}{\text{Volume (milliliters)}}$$

Specific gravity = the density of a substance relative to the density of a reference substance*.

$$\text{Specific Gravity} = \frac{\text{Density of Substance}}{\text{Density of Reference Substance}}$$

*The reference substance is usually H_2O (water), which has a density of 1 g/mL. When water is the reference substance, the specific gravity is the same value as the density but without units. For example, the density of glycerin is 1.26 g/mL. When you calculate the specific gravity of glycerin, you take the density of glycerin and divide that by the density of water (1.26 g/mL ÷ 1 g/mL = 1.26). Essentially all that happens is the units cancel out. The specific gravity of glycerin = 1.26.

EXAMPLE #1

You weigh 30 mL of a mystery substance to determine its identity. If the 30 mL sample of the substance weighs 33.3 grams, what is the identity of the substance?

A. Water (Density = 1. 0 g/mL)
B. Isopropyl Alcohol (Density = 0.79 g/mL)
C. Glycerin (Density = 1.26 g/mL)
D. Simple Syrup (Density = 1.3 g/mL)
E. Ethylene Glycol (Density = 1.11 g/mL)

SOLUTION:

$$\text{Density} = \frac{\text{Mass (g)}}{\text{Volume (mL)}} = \frac{33.3 \text{ g}}{30 \text{ mL}} = 1.11 \text{ g/mL}$$

ANSWER: E. Ethylene Glycol (Density = 1.11 g/mL)

EXAMPLE #2

To compound 60 grams of a formulation that contains 10% (w/w) petrolatum, how many milliliters of pure melted liquid petrolatum would be required? NOTE: Density of petrolatum = 0.9 g/mL

Solution:

$$\frac{10 \text{ parts of petrolatum}}{100 \text{ parts total}} \times 60 \text{ g total formulation} = 6 \text{ g of petrolatum}$$

$$6 \text{ g of petrolatum} \times \frac{\text{mL}}{0.9 \text{ g}} = 6.67 \text{ mL of petrolatum}$$

Answer: 6.67 mL of petrolatum

PRACTICE PROBLEMS

1. How much does 4 mL of a substance weigh if its density is 1.2 g/mL?

2. What volume of simple syrup (density 1.3 g/mL) would be needed to obtain a sample that weighs 2 grams?

3. What would the specific gravity of water be (density = 1 g/mL) if the reference substance was glycerin (density = 1.26 g/mL)?

4. If 78 mL of Substance H weighs 131 grams, what is the density of Substance H?

5. If 12 grams of Liquid Q occupies a volume of 15 mL, what is the specific gravity of Liquid Q (assume reference substance is water)?

PRACTICE PROBLEM ANSWERS

1. 4.8 g
2. 1.54 mL
3. 0.79
4. 1.68 g/mL
5. 0.8

TEMPERATURE CONVERSION

A temperature conversion problem will be easy points on the PTCB exam... if you know how to solve it. Memorize the equations for converting Fahrenheit to Celsius and Celsius to Fahrenheit and know how to apply them.

CONVERTING FROM FAHRENHEIT TO CELSIUS

$$°C = \frac{5}{9} \, (°F - 32)$$

CONVERTING FROM CELSIUS TO FAHRENHEIT

$$°F = \left(\frac{9}{5} \times °C\right) + 32$$

TEMPERATURE CONVERSION VALUES TO MEMORIZE

Freezing Point of Water: 0°C = 32°F
Human Body Temperature: 37°C = 98.6°F
Boiling Point of Water: 100°C = 212°F

EXAMPLE

You read that insulin should be stored at 2 – 8°C. What is this temperature range in degrees Fahrenheit?

SOLUTION:

$$\left(\frac{9}{5} \times 2°C\right) + 32 = 36°F \qquad \left(\frac{9}{5} \times 8°C\right) + 32 = 46°F$$

ANSWER: 36–46°F

PRACTICE PROBLEMS

Convert to Fahrenheit:

1) −3°C
2) 0°C
3) 1°C
4) 6°C
5) 25°C
6) 60°C

Convert to Celsius:

7) −10°F
8) 0°F
9) 32°F
10) 98.6°F
11) 72°F
12) 101°

PRACTICE PROBLEM ANSWERS

1) 27°F
2) 32°F
3) 34°F
4) 43°F
5) 77°F
6) 140°F

7) -23°C
8) -18°C
9) 0°C
10) 37°C
11) 22°C
12) 38.3°C

WEIGHT-BASED DOSING

Weight-based dosing always requires the patient's weight to be in units of kilograms (kg). Here in the United States, we typically measure a person's weight in terms of pounds, not kilograms. For this reason, converting a patient's weight from pounds to kilograms will usually be the first step in calculating a weight-based dose. A lot of problems involve converting a patient's weight from pounds to kilograms, so it is extremely important that you master this calculation. Fortunately, the calculation is simple. Just remember that 1 kg = 2.2 lbs and get a lot of practice by working through the examples and practice problems.

EXAMPLE #1

Infliximab is prescribed to a patient at a dose of 5 mg/kg. The patient weighs 154 pounds. How many milligrams of infliximab should be dispensed as one dose?

$$\frac{154 \text{ lb}}{1} \times \frac{1 \text{ kg}}{2.2 \text{ lb}} \times \frac{5 \text{ mg}}{\text{kg}} = 350 \text{ mg}$$

EXAMPLE #2

You calculate the appropriate dose of infliximab to be 350 mg. The dose is going to be administered IV in 250 mL of 0.9% NaCl. Infliximab comes in a vial containing 100 mg/20 mL solution. How many vials will you need to open in order to fill this prescription?

Answer: 4 vials (you will only use 3.5 vials, but you will need to open 4 vials since you cannot open half of a vial)

EXAMPLE #3

How many milliliters of the drug solution will be needed to obtain 350 mg of infliximab for the aforementioned prescription?

$$\frac{350 \text{ mg}}{1} \times \frac{20 \text{ mL}}{100 \text{ mg}} = 70 \text{ mL}$$

EXAMPLE #4

Vancomycin is being dosed at 15 mg/kg for a patient that weighs 241 pounds and has a fever. How many milliliters of vancomycin 1 gram/20 mL solution will be needed to compound this prescription?

$$\frac{241 \text{ lb}}{1} \times \frac{1 \text{ kg}}{2.2 \text{ lb}} \times \frac{15 \text{ mg}}{\text{kg}} \times \frac{20 \text{ mL}}{1 \text{ g}} \times \frac{1 \text{ g}}{1,000 \text{ mg}} = 32.9 \text{ mL}$$

Note: Frequently, you will receive problems that contain irrelevant information (in this case, the fact that the patient has a fever). Don't be distracted by this type of information; move on and solve the problem using the relevant information.

DOSING BASED ON BODY SURFACE AREA (BSA)

FORMULA FOR BODY SURFACE AREA (BSA)

$$BSA = \sqrt{\frac{\text{height (cm)} \times \text{weight (kg)}}{3,600}}$$

Note: Cancer chemotherapy drugs are commonly dosed according to body surface area.

EXAMPLE #1

What is the BSA of a patient that is 5 feet and 4 inches tall and weighs 110 pounds?

$$\sqrt{\frac{64 \text{ in}}{1} \times \frac{2.54 \text{ cm}}{\text{in}} \times \frac{110 \text{ lb}}{1} \times \frac{1 \text{ kg}}{2.2 \text{ lb}} \times \frac{1}{3,600}} = 1.50 \text{ m}^2$$

Note: BSA is expressed in units of square meters (m²).

EXAMPLE #2

The appropriate dose of Doxorubicin is 550 mg/m². How many milligrams are required to provide three doses to a male patient 6' 1" tall weighing 225 lbs?

$$\frac{73 \text{ in}}{1} \times \frac{2.54 \text{ cm}}{\text{in}} = 185 \text{ cm}$$

$$\frac{225 \text{ lb}}{1} \times \frac{1 \text{ kg}}{2.2 \text{ lb}} = 102 \text{ kg}$$

$$\sqrt{\frac{185 \text{ cm} \times 102 \text{ kg}}{3,600}} \times \frac{550 \text{ mg}}{\text{m}^2} \times \frac{3 \text{ doses}}{1} = 3,777 \text{ mg}$$

Note: When you convert the height and weight to the metric system separately (as demonstrated above), and then plug the numbers into the equation for BSA, your final answer will be slightly less accurate due to rounding. For this reason, it is better to perform all of the calculations at the same time (see example below).

$$\left(\sqrt{\frac{73 \text{ in}}{1} \times \frac{2.54 \text{ cm}}{\text{in}} \times \frac{225 \text{ lb}}{1} \times \frac{1 \text{ kg}}{2.2 \text{ lb}} \times \frac{1}{3,600}} \right) \times \frac{550 \text{ mg}}{\text{m}^2} \times \frac{3}{1} = 3,787 \text{ mg}$$

This answer is more accurate since the converted weight and height were not rounded.
In this case, there were only 2 significant figures, so technically, the correct answer is 3,800 mg. Both approaches yield the same answer for all practical purposes; however, it is always best to use the most accurate approach when solving math problems and then round your final answer up or down as necessary.

CALCULATING PEDIATRIC DOSES

THREE (3) METHODS FOR CALCULATING PEDIATRIC DOSES BASED ON ADULT DOSING INFORMATION

#1 Clark's Rule   #2 Young's Rule   #3 BSA dosing

CLARK'S RULE

$$\text{Child Dose} = \frac{\text{Weight (lb)}}{150 \text{ lb}} \times \text{Adult Dose}$$

What is the significance of 150 pounds?
150 pounds is the average adult weight.

Note: If the child's weight is given in kilograms, you must convert the weight to pounds. To do this, multiply the kilogram weight by the conversion factor of 2.2 pounds/kilogram.

YOUNG'S RULE

$$\text{Child Dose} = \frac{\text{Age}}{(\text{Age} + 12)} \times \text{Adult Dose}$$

Note: If the child's age is given in months, you must convert or round to the nearest year!

BSA DOSING

$$\text{Child Dose} = \frac{\text{BSA}}{1.73 \text{ m}^2} \times \text{Adult Dose}$$

What is the significance of the value 1.73 m²?
1.73 m² is the average adult body surface area (BSA).

Remember the following equation: $\text{BSA} = \sqrt{\dfrac{\text{height (cm)} \times \text{weight (kg)}}{3{,}600}}$

Note: Keep an eye on those units! Height must be in centimeters and weight must be in kilograms!

EXAMPLE #1

If dispensing a prescription for prednisone for a 6-year-old patient that is 3' 5" tall and weighs 49 pounds, what is the appropriate pediatric dose based on BSA dosing if the adult dose is 20 mg?

SOLUTION:

$$\text{Child Dose} = \frac{\sqrt{\left(\dfrac{\dfrac{41\text{ in}}{1} \times \dfrac{2.54\text{ cm}}{\text{in}} \times \dfrac{49\text{ lb}}{1} \times \dfrac{\text{kg}}{2.2\text{ lb}}}{3,600}\right)}}{1.73\text{ m}^2} \times 20\text{ mg} = 9.3\text{ mg}$$

ANSWER: 9.3 mg

EXAMPLE #2

What is the appropriate dose based on Young's Rule?

SOLUTION:

$$\text{Child Dose} = \frac{6}{(6+12)} \times 20\text{ mg} = 6.7\text{ mg}$$

ANSWER: 6.7 mg

EXAMPLE #3

What is the appropriate dose based on Clark's Rule?

SOLUTION:

$$\text{Child Dose} = \frac{49\text{ lb}}{150\text{ lb}} \times 20\text{ mg} = 6.5\text{ mg}$$

ANSWER: 6.5 mg

EXAMPLE #4

Using Clark's Rule, calculate the appropriate dose of Drug X for a 30 kg child (the adult dose is 750 mg).

A. 150 mg
B. 250 mg
C. 300 mg
D. 330 mg
E. 460 mg

SOLUTION:

$$\text{Child Dose} = \frac{\left(\frac{30\ kg}{1} \times \frac{2.2\ lb}{kg}\right)}{150\ lb} \times 750\ mg = 330\ mg$$

ANSWER: D. 330 mg

NOTE: Never overlook what units you are working with. If you forget to convert the patient's weight from kilograms to pounds before using Clark's Rule, you will miss questions like this.

PRACTICE PROBLEMS

1. The adult dose of Drug HD3021 is 400 mg once daily. What is the appropriate dose of Drug HD3021 for a 10-year-old male child that is 53 inches tall and weighs 78 pounds? Use Clark's Rule.

2. The adult dose of a drug is 150 mg twice daily for three days. How many milligrams (for a three-day course of therapy) should be dispensed to an 8-year-old female child that is 45 inches tall and weighs 57 pounds? Use Young's Rule.

3. Based on an adult dose of 600 mg, what is the appropriate dose for a 6-year-old boy that is 3 feet 4 inches tall and weighs 44 pounds? Use BSA Dosing.

4. If the adult dose of a drug is 1 gram, what is the appropriate dose for an 11-year-old child that weighs 100 pounds? Use Clark's Rule.

5. If the adult dose of a drug is 1 gram, what is the appropriate dose for an 11-year-old child that weighs 100 pounds? Use Young's Rule.

PRACTICE PROBLEM ANSWERS

1. 208 mg
2. 360 mg (60 mg per dose x 6 doses)
3. 260 mg
4. 667 mg
5. 478 mg

DRUG PRICING CALCULATIONS

Calculating drug prices is a simple process of obtaining information and entering that information into an equation. To understand the drug pricing equation, you must first understand the terms and processes by which pharmacies purchase drug products.

DRUG PURCHASING PROCESS

1. Brand and Generic Manufacturers Sell Drug Products to Wholesale Distributors*
2. Wholesale Distributors Sell Drug Products to Pharmacies
3. Pharmacies Sell Drug Products to Customers

*There are many wholesale distributors, but the largest and most well-known among them include McKesson Corporation, Cardinal Health, and AmerisourceBergen. In some cases, the pharmacy may purchase certain drug products directly from the manufacturer. See "The Role of Wholesale Distributors" below for more information.

DRUG PRICING TERMS

Average Wholesale Price (AWP)
The average price paid by a pharmacy to acquire a drug product from a wholesale distributor. Private and government insurance programs usually use AWP to calculate reimbursement rates for pharmacies.

Dispensing Fee
An amount added to the cost of each prescription dispensed by the pharmacy to cover direct and indirect costs associated with filling the prescription (e.g., employee wages, rent, and utilities). The typical dispensing fee is roughly $2 - $12 per prescription.

Markup
An amount added to the cost of a drug for resale. A markup allows the pharmacy to profit from drug sales. Most businesses mathematically define the markup as a percentage of the acquisition cost. For instance, a 20% markup means the pharmacy will make a gross profit equal to 20% of the acquisition cost of the drug.

Retail Cost
Retail Cost is the total cost of the product charged to the customer. This price does not take into account a patient's prescription drug insurance or any discount cards or coupons they may use.

Wholesale Acquisition Cost (WAC)
The list price for a drug purchased from a manufacturer by a wholesale distributor or pharmacy. Since WAC reflects the list price, WAC does not take into account any discounts or rebates that purchasers are often able to obtain.

THE ROLE OF WHOLESALE DISTRIBUTORS

You may wonder why a wholesale distributor is necessary. Why not cut out the middleman? Hundreds of drug companies manufacture thousands of products all over the globe. It would be virtually impossible for a small business, such as an independent pharmacy, to organize and manage the ordering of drug products without the help of an intermediary (a wholesale distributor); however, for the most part, large retail chains *are* able to avoid the extra expense of a wholesale distributor. They do this by setting up their own distribution system in which they fulfill drug orders using company-owned warehouses and trucks. You will hear these referred to as "warehouse orders." However, they still tend to rely on wholesale distributors for rare items, lower-cost brand name products, and/or next-day delivery.

WHERE TO OBTAIN DRUG PRICING INFORMATION

Several private companies publish up-to-date drug pricing information, but the largest and most well-known sources are:

- First DataBank
- Medi-Span
- Red Book*
- Gold Standard Drug Database

*Red Book is not to be confused with the Orange Book. The Red Book contains drug pricing information published by a private company, whereas the Orange Book is a therapeutic equivalence reference published by the federal government.

PRESCRIPTION DRUG PRICING EQUATION

Retail Cost = [AWP x (1 + Markup*)] + Dispensing Fee
*Markup expressed as a decimal

Note: There are many intricacies and complexities of drug pricing terminology. Average Wholesale Price (AWP) is a commonly used term for the drug pricing equation, but the acquisition cost can be expressed using different terms. For instance, Actual Acquisition Cost (AAC) or Wholesale Acquisition Cost (WAC). All of these terms express acquisition cost in their own way and can serve as a reasonable substitute for AWP if a value for AWP is not given.

OVER-THE-COUNTER DRUG PRICING EQUATION

Retail Cost = AWP x (1 + Markup*)
*Markup expressed as a decimal

Note: The dispensing fee does not apply to OTC drugs.

EXAMPLE #1

What is the Retail Cost (the cost to the customer) of Drug X if AWP is $49.55, the Markup is 20%, and the Dispensing Fee is $10?

Retail Cost = [AWP x (1 + Markup)] + Dispensing Fee
Retail Cost = [$49.55 x (1 + 0.2)] + $10 = $69.46

Note: If Drug X were available OTC, there would not be a dispensing fee.

EXAMPLE #2

What is the AWP for Drug Y if the Retail Cost is $9.00, the Dispensing Fee is $2.00, and the Markup is 25%?

Retail Cost = [AWP x (1 + Markup)] + Dispensing Fee
AWP = (Retail Cost – Dispensing Fee) / (1 + Markup)
AWP = ($9.00 – $2.00) / (1 + 0.25) = $7 / 1.25 = $5.60

Note: To solve this problem, we had to rearrange the equation to solve for AWP.

EXAMPLE #3

What is the Retail Cost for 30 tablets of Citalopram if the Wholesale Acquisition Cost is $6.30 for 90 tablets and the Markup on this product is 50% with a $2 Dispensing Fee?

The WAC is for 90 tablets, but our patient is only getting 30. Before entering the information into the equation, we must reduce the WAC to reflect this difference. To accomplish this, we set up a proportion because the cost of 30 tablets will be proportional to the cost of 90 tablets. In our equation, the variable "Y" represents the unknown cost of 30 tablets.

$$\frac{Y}{30 \text{ tablets}} = \frac{\$6.30}{90 \text{ tablets}}$$

Then cross multiply, and we get:

Y x 90 tablets = $6.30 x 30 tablets

Then isolate Y by dividing each side by 90 tablets:

$$Y = \frac{\$6.30 \times 30 \text{ tablets}}{90 \text{ tablets}} = \$2.10$$

Retail Cost = [WAC x (1 + Markup)] + Dispensing Fee
Retail Cost = [$2.10 x (1 + 0.50)] + $2 = $5.15

Note: In this problem, AWP is unknown; however, as we noted beneath the "Prescription Drug Pricing Equation" on the previous page, WAC is a suitable substitute for AWP when AWP is not available.

EXAMPLE #4

What is the OTC Retail Cost for a bottle of 100 caplets of acetaminophen 500 mg if the Average Wholesale Price is $2.25 and the Markup is 200%?

Retail Cost = AWP x (1 + Markup)
Retail Cost = $2.25 x (1 + 2.00) = $6.75

Note: Make sure you use the "Over-The-Counter Drug Pricing Equation" for this one and remember that only products dispensed from the pharmacy include a dispensing fee.

PRACTICE PROBLEMS

1. What is the Retail Cost of Drug B if the AWP is $20, the Dispensing Fee is $8, and the Markup is 50%?

2. What is the WAC of Drug C if the Retail Cost is $99.96, the Markup is 15%, and the Dispensing Fee is $7.50?

3. The pharmacy you work for dispenses a 30-tablet bottle of ibuprofen 800 mg for their favorite customer, Bob. The AWP is $5, the Markup is 100%, and the Dispensing Fee is $5. Bob wants to pay one-half of the Retail Cost with cash and the other half with a credit card. How much cash will Bob need?

4. What is the Retail Cost of a twin pack of OTC Robitussin if the AWP for the twin pack is $3 and the Markup is 400%?

PRACTICE PROBLEM ANSWERS

1. $38
2. $80.40
3. $7.50
4. $15

THE STEP–BY–STEP GUIDE FOR INTERPRETING PRESCRIPTION SIGS

"Sig" is short for the Latin term "signa," which means "to label." On a prescription, the sig is used by the prescriber to communicate the directions for use to the pharmacy. The pharmacy interprets the sig into plain English and places it on the label of the container that will be dispensed to the patient. In most cases, the sig on a prescription (i.e., the directions for use) will be written by the prescriber in abbreviated codes. An example would be, "take 1 tab PO BID UD," which is translated by the pharmacy to "take one tablet by mouth twice a day as directed." Many of these abbreviations are derived from Latin or Greek words. For example, BID is an abbreviation for "bis in die," which is Latin for "twice a day." A typical sig is composed of the following parts:

#1 – AN ACTION WORD
(e.g., take, give, instill, apply, place, insert, inject)

#2 – A QUANTITY WITH UNITS
(e.g., 1 tablet, 2 teaspoonsful, 4 drops, 1 gram, 1 patch, 1 suppository, 5 milliliters)

#3 – A ROUTE OF ADMINISTRATION
(e.g., by mouth, into the left eye, topically to the affected area, to the skin, rectally, vaginally, subcutaneously, intramuscularly, into each nostril, under the tongue)

#4 – THE DOSING FREQUENCY
(e.g., once daily, twice daily, three times daily, four times daily, every 2 hours, every 4 hours, every 6 hours, every 8 hours, every 12 hours, every other day, once a week, once a month)

See below for an example of a typical prescription.
Pay special attention to the sig.

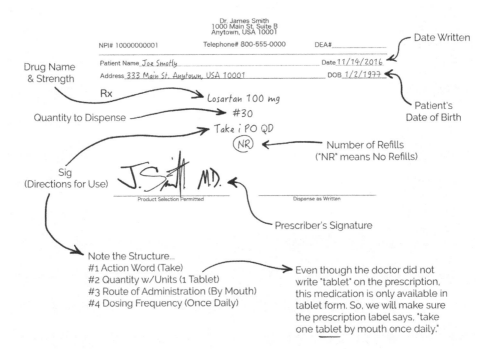

Now that you know what a sig is and what it looks like, memorize the abbreviations and complete the practice problems on the following pages to gain the knowledge and experience needed to translate sig codes.

DOSING FREQUENCIES

QOD = every other day	° = hours (e.g., Q6° = every 6 hours)
QD = every day (daily)	hs = bedtime
BID = twice daily	ac = before meals
TID = three times daily	cf = with food
QID = four times daily	wf = with food
QAM = every morning	pc = after meals
QPM = every evening	WA = while awake
Qwk = every week	ATC = around the clock
Qmo = every month	NTE = not to exceed
H = hours	PRN = as needed
D = days	STAT = immediately
SID = once daily (used only by veterinarians)	

ROUTES OF ADMINISTRATION

PO = by mouth	IVPB = intravenous piggyback
PR = rectally	IM = intramuscular
PV = vaginally	ID = intradermal
AU = both ears	IC = intracardiac
AS = left ear	IP = intraperitoneal
AD = right ear	IN = intranasal
OU = both eyes	NG = nasogastric
OS = left eye	SQ = subcutaneous
OD = right eye	SL = sublingual (under the tongue)
IV = intravenous	TD = transdermal (across the skin)
IVP = intravenous push	

DOSING INSTRUCTIONS

UD = as directed	AAA = apply to affected area

DISPENSING INSTRUCTIONS

QS = sufficient quantity
NR = no refills
DAW = dispense as written (dispense brand only)

COMPOUNDING INSTRUCTIONS

aa = of each
ad = to make; up to
div = divide
qs ad = sufficient quantity to make

SYMPTOMS AND DISEASE STATES

N/V = nausea and vomiting
HBP = high blood pressure
HTN = hypertension
BPH = benign prostatic hyperplasia (enlarged prostate)
GAD = generalized anxiety disorder
SAD = seasonal affective disorder

UNITS OF MEASURE

kg = kilogram (one thousand grams)
g = gram
mg = milligram (one one-thousandth of a gram)
μg = microgram (one one-millionth of a gram)
gr = grain (1 grain = 64.8 mg)
gtt = drop
gtts = drops
tsp = teaspoon (5 mL)
tbs = tablespoon (15 mL)
oz = ounce (one fluid ounce = 29.67 mL; one ounce of weight = 28.35 grams)
L = liter
mL = milliliter (one one-thousandth of a liter)
μL = microliter (one one-millionth of a liter)
M = molar
mM = millimolar
mEq = milliequivalent
IU = international unit

DOSAGE FORMS

cr = cream	inj = injection	CR = controlled release
crm = cream	tab = tablet	DR = delayed release
oint = ointment	cap = capsule	ER = extended release
ung = ointment	susp = suspension	LA = long acting
lot = lotion	syr = syrup	SR = sustained release
top = topical	supp = suppository	XR = extended release

STERILE COMPOUNDING ABBREVIATIONS

PPE = personal protective equipment
D5W = 5% dextrose in water
D10W = 10% dextrose in water
NSS = normal saline solution = 0.9% sodium chloride in water
½ NS = one-half normal saline = 0.45% sodium chloride in water
D5NS = 5% dextrose in normal saline
RL = Ringer's Lactate
LR = Lactated Ringers
SWFI = sterile water for injection
LVP = large volume parenteral (infusion volume greater than 100 mL)
SVP = small volume parenteral (infusion volume equal to or less than 100 mL)
MVI = multivitamin
TPN = total parenteral nutrition

MISCELLANEOUS

USP = United States Pharmacopoeia	NKA = no known allergies
NPO = nothing by mouth	NKDA = no known drug allergies
D/C = discontinue	BP = blood pressure
c̄ = with	IOP = intraocular pressure
s̄ = without	HRT = hormone replacement therapy
s̄s̄ = one-half	

ELEMENTS/LAB VALUES

Ca = calcium	K = potassium	Phos = phosphate
Cl = chloride	Mg = magnesium	Li = lithium
Fe = iron	Na = sodium	

PRACTICE PROBLEMS

1. Give s̄s̄ tsp PO cf QID x 10D

2. Inj 12 units SQ QHS

3. Insert 1 supp PR Q6H PRN

4. 1 – 2 tabs PO Q4-6H PRN severe pain

5. 1 cap PO up to Q6H PRN N/V

6. AAA on face QPM HS

7. 1 tab PO QD for HTN

8. Inj 0.25 cc IM Qmo UD

9. Instill 1 gtt OS Q2H WA

PRACTICE PROBLEM ANSWERS

1. Give one-half teaspoonful (2.5 mL) by mouth with food 4 times daily for 10 days.
2. Inject 12 units subcutaneously every night at bedtime.
3. Insert one suppository rectally every 6 hours as needed.
4. Take one to two tablets by mouth every 4 to 6 hours as needed for severe pain.
5. Take one capsule by mouth up to every 6 hours as needed for nausea and vomiting.
6. Apply to affected area on face every evening at bedtime.
7. Take one tablet by mouth once daily for hypertension.
8. Inject one-fourth mL (0.25 cc) intramuscularly every month as directed.
9. Instill one drop into left eye every two hours while awake.

COMMON DRUG NAME ABBREVIATIONS

APAP = Acetaminophen
ASA = Aspirin
CPZ = Chlorpromazine
DM = Dextromethorphan
EES = Erythromycin Ethylsuccinate
EPO = Erythropoietin
HC = Hydrocortisone
HCTZ = Hydrochlorothiazide

INH = Isoniazid
KCl = Potassium chloride
MgSO4 = Magnesium sulfate
MMI = Methimazole
MOM = Milk of Magnesia
MSO4 = Morphine sulfate
MTX = Methotrexate
NTG = Nitroglycerin
OC = Oral Contraceptive

PB = Phenobarbital
PCN = Penicillin
PE = Phenylephrine
PSE = Pseudoephedrine
PTU = Propylthiouracil
TAC = Triamcinolone
TCN = Tetracycline

NOTE: Though commonly used, it is best to avoid abbreviations due to the potential for misinterpretation.

BASIC MEDICAL TERMINOLOGY

Most English medical terms are combinations of Greek or Latin prefixes, root words, and/or suffixes. For this reason, it is in your best interest to learn the meaning of the Greek and Latin word parts used most commonly in English medical terms. See below for meanings of the most common roots, prefixes, and suffixes.

COMMON GREEK & LATIN WORD ROOTS

WORD ROOT	MEANING	EXAMPLE
Andr(o)-	Man	Androgen
Angi(o)-	Blood vessel	Angina
Arter(i)-	Artery	Arteriole
Arthr-	Joint	Arthroscopic surgery
Bio-	Life	Biohazard
Brady-	Slow	Bradycardia
Bucc-	Cheek	Buccal lozenge
Carcin-	Cancerous	Carcinoma
Cardi-	Heart	Cardiologist
Derm-	Skin	Dermatologist
Enter-	Intestines	Enteric-coated tablets
Gastr-	Stomach	Gastroesophageal reflux
Gen(esis)	Produce, generate	Genetic
Gluco-	Sweet	Glucose
Glyc-	Sugar	Hyperglycemia
Isch-	Restriction	Ischemic heart disease
Hem(at)-	Blood	Hematology
Hepat-	Liver	Hepatoma
Lip(o)-	Fat	Liposuction
My(o)-	Muscle	Myelitis
Narc(o)-	Numb, stupor	Narcotic
Nas(o)-	Nose	Nasal spray
Nephr-	Kidney	Nephrology
Neur-	Nerve	Neurology
Ocul-	Eye	Ocular
Onc-	Tumor	Oncology
Ophthalm-	Eye	Ophthalmology
Oste-	Bone	Osteomyelitis
Ot-	Ear	Otic
Path-	Disease	Pathology
Pharmaco-	Drug	Pharmacotherapy
Phren-	The mind	Schizophrenic
Plasia-	Development	Hyperplasia
Poro-	Porous	Osteoporosis
Proct(o)-	Anus, rectum	Proctologist
Psych-	Mind	Psychosis
Pyr(o)-	Fever	Antipyretic
Ren-	Kidney	Renal
Rhin-	Nose	Allergic rhinitis
Schiz(o)-	Split	Schizoid
Scler-	Hard	Atherosclerosis
Tachy-	Fast	Tachycardia
Thromb-	Clot	Thrombosis
Ur-	Urine	Nocturia
Vas(o)-	Blood vessel	Vasodilation

COMMON GREEK & LATIN PREFIXES

PREFIX	MEANING	EXAMPLE
Ante-	Before	Ante room
Anti-	Against, opposed to	Antiepileptic
Di-	Two	Dihydrogen monoxide
Heter(o)-	Different	Heterogeneous
Hom(o)-	Same	Homogeneous
Hyper-	Over, above	Hypertension
Hyp(o)-	Under, below	Hypotension
Micro-	Millionth	Microgram
Milli-	Thousandth	Milligram
Mono-	Single, one	Monoxide
Poly-	Many	Polypharmacy
Post-	After	Post-traumatic stress

COMMON GREEK & LATIN SUFFIXES

SUFFIX	MEANING	EXAMPLE
-al	Pertaining to	Intestinal
-algia	Pain	Myalgia
-ase	Enzyme	HMG CoA Reductase
-asis	Condition	Psoriasis
-emia	Blood condition	Leukemia
-emesis	Vomiting	Hyperemesis
-ia	State, condition	Hypokalemia
-iac	Pertaining to	Cardiac
-ic	Pertaining to	Prostatic hyperplasia
-ical	Pertaining to	Biological
-ion	Process	Dilution
-ism	Process, condition	Hypothyroidism
-itis	Inflammation	Arthritis
-lepsy	Attack, seizure	Epilepsy
-logy	The study of	Anesthesiology
-oid	Resembling	Opioid
-oma	Tumor	Sarcoma
-ose	Carbohydrate	Sucrose
-osis	Abnormal condition	Ketoacidosis
-ous	Pertaining to	Gangrenous
-penia	Deficiency	Leukopenia
-rrhea	Discharge	Diarrhea
-rrhage	Burst, excessive flow	Hemorrhage
-tension	Pressure	Hypertension
-tensive	Pressure	Hypotensive
-tic	Pertaining to	Neurotic

COMMON MEDICAL TERMS

Absorption – the movement of a drug from a delivery medium (e.g., tablet, capsule, transdermal patch) into the bloodstream.

Acute – a sudden or rapidly occurring symptom or condition, usually of an urgent nature. Opposite of chronic.

ADME – an acronym that stands for "Absorption, Distribution, Metabolism, and Elimination," which is the order by which drugs enter and exit the body.

Adrenal Gland – an anatomical structure located above each kidney that secretes several hormones, including cortisol, aldosterone, epinephrine, and norepinephrine.

Adrenergic – pertaining to neurons that release epinephrine or norepinephrine. Epinephrine and norepinephrine are associated with the fight or flight response.

Agonist – a substance that stimulates an action. For example, adrenaline (or "epinephrine") is an alpha and beta-receptor agonist. By stimulating these receptors, adrenaline elevates heart rate and blood pressure.

Analgesic – a drug that reduces pain.

Anaphylaxis – a severe, potentially life-threatening allergic reaction.

Anesthetic – a drug that induces partial or complete loss of sensation.

Angina – severe chest pain caused by insufficient blood flow to the heart.

Angiotensin Converting Enzyme – a key catalyst in the body that is involved in the production and release of blood pressure-raising hormones.

Antacid – a drug that neutralizes stomach acid.

Antagonist – a drug that opposes an action. For example, metoprolol is a beta-receptor antagonist ("beta blocker"). Metoprolol interferes with the stimulation of beta-receptors, thereby opposing increases in heart rate and blood pressure.

Antiarrhythmic – a drug that treats or prevents cardiac arrhythmias.

Antibiotic – a drug that kills or opposes the reproduction of microorganisms.

Anticholinergic – a drug that opposes parasympathetic nervous system activity. The parasympathetic nervous system is associated with rest and digestion.

Anticoagulant – a drug that treats or prevents blood clots.

Anticonvulsant – a substance or medication that prevents or treats seizures.

Antidepressant – a drug that treats or prevents mental depression.

Antidiabetic – a drug that lowers blood sugar levels.

Antidiarrheal – a drug that treats or prevents diarrhea.

Antidote – a drug that neutralizes a poison or opposes the effect of a poison.

Antiemetic – a drug that treats or prevents nausea and vomiting.

Antiepileptic – a drug that treats or prevents epilepsy or seizures. Often used synonymously with the term "anticonvulsant."

Antifungal – a drug that kills or interferes with the reproduction of fungi.

Antihistamine – prevents the release or blocks the action of histamine, a mediator of allergic reactions, stomach acid production, and mental alertness/wakefulness.

Antiplatelet – a drug that opposes the activity of platelets. Platelets play a major role in blood clot formation.

Antipsychotic – a drug that treats or prevents psychosis (e.g., bipolar disorder, schizophrenia).

Antipyretic – a drug that reduces fever.

Antitussive – a drug that suppresses a cough.

Antiviral – a drug that treats viral infections.

Arteries – blood vessels that carry oxygenated blood from the heart to the organs.

Atherosclerosis – hardening and occlusion of arteries caused by the build-up of calcium and cholesterol.

Atrial Fibrillation – a type of cardiac arrhythmia in which a specific area of the heart (the right atrium) receives irregular electrical impulses from the nervous system, causing a rapid, irregular heartbeat. This irregular heartbeat can cause blood clots capable of traveling to the brain and causing strokes. Abbreviations for atrial fibrillation include "AF" and "A-fib."

Benign Prostatic Hyperplasia (BPH) – non-cancerous growth/enlargement of the prostate gland. The enlarged prostate presses against the urethra, blocking the outflow of urine.

Blood Glucose – a measure of the concentration of glucose (sugar) in the blood. High blood glucose (see "hyperglycemia") is a sign of diabetes.

Blood Clot – a mass of coagulated blood capable of blocking blood flow.
Bradycardia – below normal heart rate. (Normal resting heart rate is 60-90 beats per minute.)

Cardiac Arrhythmia – any condition in which the heart beats irregularly (e.g., beats off rhythm, beats too fast, beats too slow).

Cardiovascular System – an organ system composed of the heart and the blood vessels (arteries and veins).

Ceiling Effect – a phenomenon where the therapeutic effect increases only up to a certain point (the "ceiling"). Higher doses impart no additional benefit, causing additional side effects without increasing the therapeutic effect.

Cholesterol – a fatty substance the body uses to produce hormones and cell walls. Excess cholesterol accumulates in arterial blood vessels, causing atherosclerosis and increasing the risk of a heart attack.

Cholinergic – a drug that produces or mimics the effects of acetylcholine.

Chronic – a symptom or condition that worsens slowly over time, sometimes progressing undetected. The opposite of acute.

Contraceptive – a drug or device that prevents conception/pregnancy.

Coronary Artery Disease (CAD) – narrowing of the arteries that supply blood to the heart, typically caused by atherosclerosis.

Corticosteroid – an anti-inflammatory drug that mimics the hormone "cortisol" which is produced by the adrenal gland. Examples include hydrocortisone and prednisone.

Decongestant – a drug that reduces nasal congestion.

Depressant – a drug that decreases nerve activity, potentially to the point of sedation.

Diuresis – increased urine production. Diuretic drugs (loop diuretics, thiazide diuretics, and potassium-sparing diuretics) work by inducing diuresis.

Edema – swelling. Treatment for edema usually involves a loop diuretic.

Electrolytes – electrically charged minerals. Examples include potassium, calcium, and sodium. Electrolytes are essential for normal body function (e.g., muscle contraction and nerve function).

Elimination – the physiologic removal of a product from the body. In many cases, the liver metabolizes and deactivates a drug and then the kidneys transfer the waste product into the urine for elimination.

Embolism – obstruction of a blood vessel by some form of debris or a foreign body. For example, a blood clot, a mass of cholesterol, or an air bubble.

Emesis – vomiting.

Enzyme – a catalyst for a chemical reaction. The body naturally produces certain enzymes.

Epistaxis – nosebleed.

Expectorant – a drug that thins mucus, making it easier to expel/cough up.

Glaucoma – a disease characterized by increased intraocular pressure.

Gout – a disease characterized by severe joint pain and inflammation.

Heart Failure – a condition in which the heart is unable to pump forcefully or effectively enough to meet the needs of the body.

Hepatic – pertaining to the liver.

Histamine – a substance produced within the body that, when released, elicits symptoms associated with allergic reactions, such as a runny nose, itchy/watery eyes, and rashes. Histamine also plays a role in stomach acid production and mental alertness/wakefulness.

HMG-CoA Reductase – the key enzyme involved in hepatic cholesterol production.

Hormone – a substance produced by the body to regulate or stimulate certain physiologic functions. Examples of hormones include insulin, estrogen, progesterone, and testosterone.

Hyperglycemia – abnormally high level of glucose in the blood.

Hyperkalemia – abnormally high level of potassium in the blood.

Hypertension – high blood pressure.

Hyperuricemia – abnormally high uric acid levels in the blood.

Hypoglycemia – abnormally low level of glucose in the blood.

Hypokalemia – abnormally low level of potassium in the blood.

Hypotension – low blood pressure.

Indication – a use for a drug; a condition or symptom for which a drug is effective in treating. For example, hypertension is an indication for lisinopril.

Lacrimation – the production of tears.

Lipids – fats.

Metabolism – the body's natural process of chemically altering or breaking down a substance (e.g., a drug) with the goal of removing the substance from the body.

Myocardial Infarction (MI) – an event in which a portion of heart muscle tissue dies due to occlusion of the coronary artery.

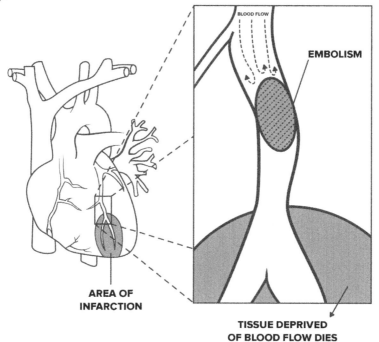

Nephron – the most basic unit of the kidney. Diuretic drugs work by modulating electrolyte exchange at certain locations in the nephron; for example, loop diuretics prevent sodium from being re-absorbed from the Loop of Henle (a segment of the nephron).

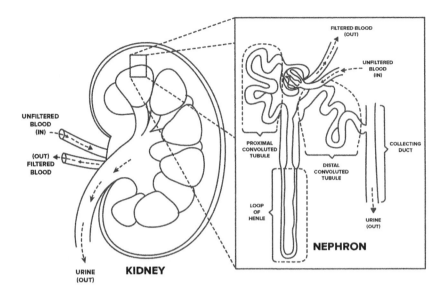

Neuron – a nerve cell; the most basic unit of the nervous system.

Neurotransmitter – a substance released by neurons to manage nervous system-mediated functions. One example is serotonin, which helps manage behavior and mood.

Nitric Oxide – a chemical in the body that causes blood vessels to dilate/expand.

Nonproductive Cough – dry cough.

Non-Steroidal Anti-Inflammatory Drugs (NSAIDs) – medications that work similar to corticosteroids, reducing pain and swelling caused by inflammation.

Off-Label – a term that describes uses for a drug that are not FDA-approved.

Osmosis – the process by which water naturally crosses a semipermeable membrane from the side with low solute concentration to the side with a high solute concentration in an attempt to equalize the solute concentration on each side of the membrane.

Parenteral – Administered by a route other than the gastrointestinal tract.

Peripheral Neuropathy – tingling or pain in the extremities caused by nerve damage.

Phosphodiesterase-5 (PDE-5) – a key enzyme involved in the breakdown of nitric oxide.

Photosensitivity – increased sensitivity to sunlight, resulting in a predisposition to sunburn.

Polyuria – excessive urine production.

Pregnancy Category – a rating that summarizes the risk of using of a particular drug during pregnancy. The pregnancy categories are A, B, C, D, and X, where "A" is the least likely to cause birth defects, and "X" is the most likely to cause birth defects. Pregnant women should never use a drug with a pregnancy category X rating. The use of a pregnancy category A, B, C, or D drug during pregnancy may be appropriate if the benefits outweigh the risks.

Priapism – a painful, prolonged erection.

Prophylaxis – a measure or action taken to prevent disease. Synonymous with "prevention."

Prostaglandins – a group of chemicals naturally produced and released within the body for various functions, including the promotion of inflammation.

QT Interval – the time between the Q-wave and T-wave on an electrocardiogram. Some drugs can prolong the QT interval, potentially causing life-threatening cardiac arrhythmias.

EKG OF A NORMAL HEARTBEAT

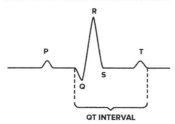

Renal – pertaining to the kidney (e.g., "renal failure" and "kidney failure" are synonymous). The kidneys function as a filtration system for blood.

Sedative-Hypnotic – a drug that induces sleep. Also referred to as tranquilizer.

Serotonin Syndrome – a condition caused by excessive stimulation of serotonin receptors.

Side Effects – the undesired effects/consequences of medication use.

Solute – a drug that is dissolved in a solution.

Solution – the liquid that contains a dissolved drug; a homogeneous mixture composed of a solute and a solvent.

Solvent – the liquid part of a solution in which the solute is dissolved.

Stevens-Johnson syndrome (SJS) – a disease characterized by fever and severe skin rashes involving the mouth, eyes, and mucous membranes.

Stimulant – a drug that increases nerve activity.

Stroke – an event in which an area of the brain dies due to insufficient blood flow.

Sulfa Allergy – an allergy to the class of antibiotics known as the sulfonamides.

Symptom – a sign that indicates the presence of a medical condition, disease, or disorder. For example, a sore throat, nasal congestion, mild fever, sneezing, and cough are all symptoms of the common cold.

Syncope – pass out; faint.

Tachycardia – abnormally rapid resting heart rate. (Normal resting heart rate is 60-90 beats per minute)

Tolerance – decreased sensitivity to a drug; the acquired capacity to endure large doses with minimal effects.

Vasoconstrictor – a drug that causes contraction/narrowing of a blood vessel, decreasing the volume of blood flowing through the vessel and increasing blood pressure.

Vasodilator – a drug that causes expansion/relaxation of a blood vessel, which increases the volume of blood flowing through the vessel and decreases blood pressure.

Veins – blood vessels that carry deoxygenated blood from the organs back to the heart.

Withdrawal – response to discontinuation of a drug to which a person has become physically or psychologically dependent.

DRUG ADMINISTRATION EQUIPMENT AND SUPPLIES

Medicine cup – Reasonably accurate for measuring in one teaspoonful (5 mL) intervals. Not accurate enough for smaller measurements.

Calibrated spoon – Used to measure and administer liquid medications when the volume to be measured is between 1–10 mL. The spoon-shaped opening makes it potentially useful for use with pediatric and geriatric patients.

Dropper – Used to measure and administer very small amounts of liquid medication (e.g., fluoride drops, infant vitamins). Typically supplied with the medication from the manufacturer and may be calibrated to measure in a variety of units depending on the medication. Usually employed for measurements of 2 mL or less.

Oral syringe – Used to make precise measurements, usually down to the tenth of a milliliter, for oral administration (not for injection). The most common oral syringes are designed to hold up to 1, 5, or 10 mL.

Tablet cutter (or pill splitter) – Device with a safety-guarded steel blade designed to cut tablets into even halves.

Spacer – A tube-like chamber with an opening at each end. One end attaches to an inhaler (e.g., an albuterol inhaler), and the patient places their mouth around the other end. The medication enters the spacer, which holds the aerosolized drug until the patient inhales through the other end. Spacers are particularly useful for patients who may have poor coordination (e.g., pediatric and geriatric patients).

Nebulizer – A device that delivers compressed air through a tube and into a special cup that turns nebulizer solution (a specially-designed liquid medication) into a mist that the patient can inhale to treat various types of lung disease (e.g., asthma, COPD, cystic fibrosis).

Lancet – A small sterile needle designed to poke a tiny hole in the skin to obtain a small blood sample, commonly used for blood glucose testing in patients with diabetes. A lancet should always be disposed of properly in a sharps container and should never be reused.

Lancing device – A typically spring-loaded device designed to penetrate the skin with a pre-loaded lancet at the push of a button.

Blood glucose test strips – A small, rectangular piece of material that is specifically designed to collect a small amount of blood (after creating a tiny hole in the skin with a lancet) to be analyzed with a blood glucose meter.

Blood glucose meter (or glucometer) – A compact electronic device that measures the concentration of glucose (sugar) in the blood collected on a blood glucose test strip.

Insulin syringe – Designed specifically for the measurement and administration of insulin. Calibrated to measure in terms of insulin units where 1 mL is equal to 100 units of standard insulin. Most common size is 1 mL; however, smaller sizes are available (i.e., 0.5 mL and 0.3 mL).

Pen needles – An injection needle with a plastic hub that is designed to be attached to various types of injection pens (e.g., insulin pens). Many patients prefer self-injecting medications using injection pens and pen needles because they are much easier to use compared to drawing up the medication from a vial and injection with a syringe.

Standard syringe – May be used to administer injections by various routes (e.g., intravenous, intramuscular). The most commonly used size for administering injections is 3 mL. Larger capacity syringes are commercially available (e.g., 5–60 mL); however, they are typically used for sterile compounding, not for administering injections. See the next page for an illustration.

ANATOMY OF A STANDARD SYRINGE & NEEDLE

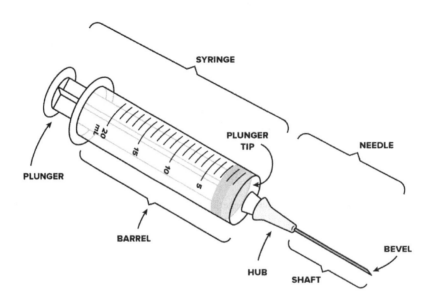

NEEDLE GAUGE SIZE

30-Gauge Needle   16-Gauge Needle

KEY POINT: Gauge size is inversely proportional to the diameter of the needle lumen.
In other words, the higher the gauge, the thinner the needle.

NDC NUMBERS

A National Drug Code (NDC) number is an 11-digit number composed of three parts. The first part identifies who manufactured the product, the second part identifies what the product is, and the third part typically identifies the size of the package or the quantity of dosage units contained in the package. The standard format of an NDC number is as follows:

$$12345–1234–12$$

First Segment (five digits)
The first segment of an NDC number identifies the manufacturer of the product (e.g., 00093 is the 5-digit code for TEVA and 52544 is the five-digit code for Watson Pharmaceuticals).

Second Segment (four digits)
The middle segment of an NDC number identifies the product made by the manufacturer (e.g., 0913 is Watson Pharmaceutical's four-digit code for Norco® 5/325 mg).

Third Segment (two digits)
The last segment of an NDC number usually identifies the package size of the product (e.g., the NDC number for a 100-tablet bottle of Watson Pharmaceutical's Norco® 5/325 mg is 52544-0913-01; whereas, the NDC number for a 500-tablet bottle is 52544-0913-05).

Note: In most cases, a leading zero is omitted from the NDC number displayed on the label of the manufacturer's stock bottle. For instance, the 11-digit NDC 00093-0287-01 would typically be displayed in one of the following three 10-digit formats:

0093-0287-01
00093-287-01
00093-0287-1

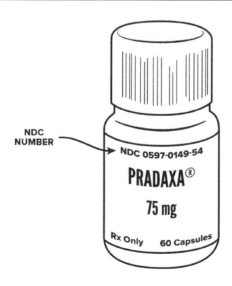

LOT NUMBERS AND EXPIRATION DATES

Are all drug products required to possess a lot number?
Yes, all drug products must have a lot number displayed on the package label.

What are lot numbers, and why are they important?
The lot number is a unique identifier consisting of a series of numbers and/or letters as assigned by the manufacturer. Manufacturers produce drug products in large batches, and the lot number identifies the batch from which the contents of that container originated. Lot numbers play a crucial role in recalls. If a manufacturer distributes a drug product to pharmacies and subsequently discovers an abnormality, such as discoloration or contamination, then they will recall the affected batch. Pharmacies use the lot number to identify and remove the recalled product from their inventory, thus preventing distribution to patients.

What happens if a drug product has no lot number (e.g., the label is damaged, and the lot number is illegible)?
Containers of a recalled drug with no lot number must be treated as though they have been recalled.

Are all prescription drugs required to have an expiration date?
Yes, the FDA requires manufacturers to assign expiration dates for all prescription drugs.

Is it acceptable to use or dispense a drug product that is expired?
No. The expiration date is the final date through which the manufacturer can guarantee the potency and safety of the drug.

If a drug product has an expiration date of 08/2024, will the product be "expired" on 08/02/2024?
No, the drug will be expired on the final day of 08/2024, which would be 08/31/2024.

What is unique about the expiration date for a vial of insulin?
Depending on the formulation, a vial of insulin may be used for up to 28 days (e.g., NovoLog®, Lantus®) or 42 days (e.g., Novolin® R, Novolin® N, Levemir®) after the rubber stopper has been punctured or until the expiration date printed on the vial, whichever comes first.

EXAMPLE

The date is July 14, 2016. You are working as a pharmacy technician in a hospital, and a nurse asks you, "When do I have to throw away this vial of NovoLog®?" The expiration date printed on the vial reads "EXP: 09/31/2021," but the nurse informs you that she initially opened the vial on July 1, 2021. What is the last day this vial of insulin can be used?

    A. 07/14/2021
    B. 07/29/2021
    C. 07/30/2021
    D. 09/31/2021

Answer: Since insulin comes in a multi-dose vial, we must assign a beyond-use date equal to 28 days from the date of first use. For that reason, choice "B" is correct.

Note: Periodically (e.g., monthly), pharmacy personnel must check each item in the pharmacy's inventory to remove any expired products. Furthermore, each time a new shipment of medication is added to the shelf, the pharmacy technician must "rotate the stock." In other words, move the older items toward the front edge of the shelf and place the new items in the back. This helps to ensure that the older medications are dispensed sooner, reducing the chance of accumulating expired medications. Expired medications are ineffective, potentially unsafe, and cannot be dispensed.

DRUG AND SUPPLY RETURNS

FDA POLICY

According to a policy from the U.S. Food and Drug Administration (FDA), unused (or partially used) prescription drugs should not be returned after leaving the pharmacy. This policy exists to protect public health. After a medication has left the pharmacy, the pharmacist can no longer supervise the conditions under which the medications are stored, and, consequently, there exists a possibility that the strength, quality, purity, and/or identity of the product has been compromised. To reinforce this policy and further attempt to protect the public health, several state boards of pharmacy also forbid the return of prescription drugs after leaving the pharmacy.

NOTE: If the pharmacist accepted a returned prescription from a patient and subsequently re-dispensed any portion of the returned drug, she would be legally liable for any issues related to adulteration or contamination. The FDA has seen cases where injuries were caused by medications that were returned and re-dispensed.

RETURN TO STOCK

"Return to stock" occurs when a drug is returned for re-dispensing. Prescription drugs may be returned to the pharmacy shelves for re-dispensing (i.e., returned to stock) in the following situations: #1 The prescription has been filled (or is in the process of being filled) and the patient either has not arrived to purchase the prescription or indicates he does not want the prescription. #2 The patient purchases the prescription but decides while remaining at the pharmacy counter (and under the supervision of the pharmacist) that he does not actually want or need the prescription. In both cases, the medication does not leave the premises or the supervision of the pharmacist.

CREDIT RETURN

A medication (or supply) is returned to the wholesaler, and a refund is issued to the pharmacy's account in the form of a credit toward future purchases. It is important to follow the procedures of the wholesaler to ensure credit can be obtained for the return. For a product to be eligible for credit, unless it was somehow defective, the wholesaler will typically require the medication to be in its original sealed container, and the pharmacist must attest that the medication has been stored under the appropriate conditions (e.g., temperature).

EXPIRED MEDICATIONS

Expired medications cannot be dispensed. Each pharmacy must create and follow a policy for identifying and removing expired medications and supplies from stock. As an example, a pharmacy may assign each technician to check all of the items stocked in a specific area of the pharmacy every 30 days and remove from the shelves any medications or supplies that are expired ("outdated") or about to expire ("short-dated") and place them in a separate area designated for removal.

REVERSE DISTRIBUTION

Reverse distributors are entities that accept unusable, unwanted, or expired products from pharmacies and assist with acquiring manufacturer or wholesaler credits for resalable products and with managing the disposal process for non-creditable products.

PHARMACY TECHNICIAN CERTIFICATION
SUMMARY OF RENEWAL REQUIREMENTS

- Once certified, recertification is required every 2 years
- Obtain 20 hours of continuing education (CE) in each 2-year recertification cycle
    - Subject matter must be pharmacy-technician specific
    - At least 1 hour on the subject of pharmacy law
    - At least 1 hour on the subject of patient safety
    - Keep CE participation certificates as evidence of completion*
- Apply for recertification online at PTCB.org
    - Must pay a $49 recertification fee

*The PTCB may randomly select pharmacy technicians to audit their continuing education credits. For that reason, it is important to keep participation certificates as evidence of continuing education completion.

CONGRATULATIONS!

Congratulations! You are almost prepared to take the PTCB exam. Don't quit until you feel 100% confident. Be sure to memorize as much as possible. Only *you* can accurately judge your level of readiness. Once you're finished with this study guide, test your knowledge and skills with our full-length practice exam that begins on the next page.

Final thoughts...
- If you have never been to the testing center where your exam is scheduled, travel there a few days prior to the exam so you know how to get there and what to expect in terms of parking (if applicable).
- Try to be well-rested, well-hydrated, and well-fed on exam day.
- Do not rush through the exam.
- If you begin to panic, take a deep breath, and remember that failure is not fatal.
- The test is multiple-choice, so if you don't know the right answer, then rule out the obvious wrong answers before taking a guess. There is no penalty for guessing.
- Don't select answers you have never heard of when guessing (e.g., if you have it narrowed down to "A. Diabetes" or "B. Diffuse Intravascular Coagulation," then choose "A. Diabetes"). The answer is probably easier than you think.
- As I've pointed out several times now, the entire exam is multiple-choice (including the math problems). Usually, multiple-choice exams benefit the test-taker, but be careful! When math problems are presented in a multiple-choice format, the various choices can be designed to trick and deceive you. My advice for math problems is to solve them and double-check your answer with a calculator **before** looking at the answer options.
- Remember, you get 110 minutes (1 hour and 50 minutes) to complete the exam, and you need a scaled score of 1400 to pass (note the possible score range: 1000–1600). That means you have to get about 70% of the questions correct. The practice exam on the pages that follow contains 90 questions, just like the official PTCB exam. For the purposes of this practice exam, assume each problem is worth one point. For answers that are completely or partially wrong, you do not receive the point. When you are finished, add up all of your points and divide that number by 90. You will get a decimal (something between 0.00 and 1.00). Multiply that number by 100%. For instance, if you answered 80 of the questions correctly, you would divide 80 by 90, which equals 0.89. Multiply 0.89 by 100%. That equals 89%. An 89% would be an example of a passing score (> 70%).
- One last thing. The practice exam answer key (on pages 226-237) was created to function as a teaching tool. I didn't just throw the answers back there. Each answer in the answer key is accompanied by a detailed explanation and/or an exact reference to the page(s) you can turn to for a quick review of the relevant content. I highly encourage you to read the entire answer key after completing the practice exam. It will go a long way toward helping you prepare for the real thing.

Proceed with confidence!
David A Heckman, PharmD

PRACTICE EXAM

SET A TIMER FOR 1 HOUR AND 50 MINUTES

THEN PROCEED

1. Mr. Tucker weighs 65 kg. What is Mr. Tucker's weight in pounds?

    A. 65 lb
    B. 130 kg
    C. 143 lb
    D. 154 lb

2. If a bottle of Protonix® has a manufacturer-assigned expiration date of 09/2022, what is the last day it can be used?

    A. August 31, 2022
    B. September 1, 2022
    C. September 30, 2022
    D. October 1, 2022
    E. None of the above

3. What is the generic drug name for Keppra®?

    A. Lansoprazole
    B. Lamotrigine
    C. Ipratropium
    D. Levetiracetam

4. Which insulin formulation(s) is/are considered to be "rapid acting?"

    A. NovoLog®
    B. Levemir®
    C. Apidra®
    D. Both A & B
    E. Both A & C

5. What is the route of administration for Xalatan® (Latanoprost)?

    A. Otic
    B. Ophthalmic
    C. Oral
    D. Topical
    E. Rectal

6. Which drug class is associated with the side effect of dry, nonproductive cough?

    A. Beta Blockers
    B. Angiotensin Receptor Blockers
    C. HMG-CoA Reductase Inhibitors
    D. Serotonin-Norepinephrine Reuptake Inhibitors
    E. Angiotensin Converting Enzyme Inhibitors

7. A patient who takes Coumadin® is more likely to experience bleeding problems when taking which of these medications? (Select all that apply)

    ☐ aspirin
    ☐ naproxen
    ☐ Augmentin®
    ☐ ciprofloxacin
    ☐ clindamycin

8. Match each brand name with the correct generic name.

A. Singulair®   I. Phenytoin
B. Desyrel®   II. Benzonatate
C. Dilantin®   III. Diazepam
D. Tessalon®   IV. Trazodone
E. Valium®   V. Montelukast

9. Match each drug with its corresponding indication.

A. Meloxicam   I. Insomnia
B. Fexofenadine II. Pain
C. Olmesartan   III. Inflammation
D. Fentanyl   IV. Hypertension
E. Zolpidem   V. Allergies

10. Which agency is responsible for enforcing the federal Controlled Substances Act?

A. FDA
B. DEA
C. OSHA
D. FTC
E. None of the above

11. Which controlled substance schedule fits the following description?

"Includes drugs that are used medically but have a high potential for abuse and physical/psychological dependence."

A. Schedule I
B. Schedule II
C. Schedule III
D. Schedule IV
E. Schedule V

12. What is the name of the form used to order Schedule II controlled substances?

A. DEA Form 41
B. DEA Form 222
C. Invoice
D. DEA Form 106
E. Pharmacy C-II Order Sheet

13. Pill counting trays and countertops should be cleaned at least once daily using _____.

A. Soap and warm water
B. 1:10 mixture of bleach and sterile water
C. 70% isopropyl alcohol
D. None of the above

14. Adverse events related to which of the following should not be reported to the FDA through MedWatch?

    A. Prescription Drugs
    B. Over the Counter Drugs
    C. Vaccines
    D. None of the above

15. What is the name of the REMS program for isotretinoin?

    A. T.I.P.S.
    B. S.T.E.P.S.
    C. iPLEDGE
    D. Clozaril National Registry
    E. The Isotretinoin Damage Prevention Program

16. What is the maximum amount of pseudoephedrine one person may purchase in one day?

    A. 2 grams
    B. 3.6 grams
    C. 7.5 grams
    D. 9 grams
    E. 5 boxes

17. Which of the following anxiety medications is not a Schedule IV controlled substance?

    A. Alprazolam
    B. Buspirone
    C. Clonazepam
    D. Diazepam

18. Which of the following is not an error-prone abbreviation?

    A. QD
    B. QOD
    C. OD
    D. All of the above are error-prone abbreviations

19. Which antibiotic is only available for topical use?

    A. Mupirocin
    B. Cefdinir
    C. Azithromycin
    D. Doxycycline
    E. Metronidazole

20. What is wrong with the prescription shown below?

James Smith, D.O.
Simplified Medical Clinic
10001 N. Main St. Suite 100A, Simple City, USA 24680
Telephone# 123-555-1234

Name _Jane Doe_   Age _44_

Address _555 South Main St. Anywhere, USA 10001_   Date _3/30/20_

Rx

Norco 5/325 mg tablets

60 (sixty)

Take i-ii PO Q4-6H PRN for pain

| NR | (1) | 2 | 3 | 4 | 5 | PRN |

James Smith , D.O.

Prescriber must write "Brand Medically Necessary" on the prescription to prohibit generic substitution.

A. Refills cannot be issued for Norco® because it is a Schedule II controlled substance
B. The patient's state-issued ID number is not written on the prescription
C. The prescriber's DEA number is not written on the prescription
D. Both A & C
E. All of the above

21. Which of the following is done to identify the underlying cause of a dispensing error?

    A. Separate inventory
    B. Root-cause analysis
    C. Tall man lettering
    D. Action plan

22. Which antihistamine can be used to treat anxiety?

    A. Cetirizine
    B. Fexofenadine
    C. Hydroxyzine
    D. Loratadine

23. Which sig code is not an error-prone abbreviation according to the Institute for Safe Medication Practices (ISMP)?

    A. HS (bedtime)
    B. SQ (subcutaneous)
    C. PO (by mouth)
    D. IU (international units)

24. You are using a class A prescription balance with a sensitivity requirement of 6 mg. With this balance, you are able to measure 300 mg of a substance within ___ % error.

    A. 1
    B. 2
    C. 3
    D. 4
    E. 5

25. You receive an order for 90 milliliters of lidocaine 4% nasal spray. You will use normal saline solution and 10% lidocaine solution to compound this prescription. How much 10% lidocaine solution will be needed?

    A. 18 mL
    B. 27 mL
    C. 36 mL
    D. 45 mL
    E. 54 mL

26. A patient presents a prescription for 450 milliliters of allopurinol 40 mg/mL oral suspension. Allopurinol is available from the manufacturer only as an oral tablet. Using allopurinol 100 mg tablets, how many tablets will you need to pulverize and triturate to compound this prescription?

    A. 90 tablets
    B. 100 tablets
    C. 125 tablets
    D. 180 tablets
    E. 250 tablets

27. Hydralazine and Hydroxyzine are examples of _____.

    A. Allergy medications
    B. Brand name medications
    C. Separating inventory
    D. Look-alike/sound-alike medications
    E. Drug regimen reviews

28. Humalog® and NovoLog® are examples of _____.

    A. Rapid acting insulin
    B. Brand name medications
    C. High-alert medications
    D. All of the above
    E. None of the above

29. What is the purpose of tall man lettering?

    A. To emphasize the differences in spelling between medications with similar names.
    B. To standardize the font size for medication names as they appear on stock bottles.
    C. To make it easier to separate inventory.
    D. To eliminate the need for NDC numbers.
    E. None of the above.

30. How does the use of leading zeros affect the likelihood of a prescription order interpretation error?

    A. The use of leading zeros increases the likelihood of an error.
    B. The use of leading zeros decreases the likelihood of an error.
    C. The use of leading zeros does not affect the likelihood of an error.
    D. It depends on the identity of the patient.

31. Which situation requires pharmacist intervention?

    A. Receiving a prescription from a new patient.
    B. Answering the telephone.
    C. Counting tablets to fill a prescription for amlodipine.
    D. Recommending an over the counter medication for a patient.
    E. All of the above.

32. Why are anticoagulants, such as heparin and warfarin, considered to be "high-alert" medications?

    A. Because they have a caffeine-like effect.
    B. Because over 20% of patients are allergic to anticoagulants.
    C. Because excessive doses can cause severe and potentially fatal bleeding.
    D. Because overdoses can cause hypoglycemia.

33. Which employee(s) is/are authorized to perform a drug utilization review (DUR)?

    A. Pharmacy Technician
    B. Certified Pharmacy Technician
    C. Pharmacist
    D. Cashier
    E. Both B & C

34. Which two entities are working together in a campaign to eliminate the use of error-prone abbreviations?

    A. FDA and DEA
    B. FBI and CIA
    C. WHO and OSHA
    D. ISMP and FDA
    E. IRS and FDIC

35. For a physician to prescribe Suboxone® outside of a narcotic treatment facility, he must have a special DEA number that begins with which letter?

    A. A
    B. F
    C. X
    D. Y
    E. Z

36. Which of the following could be an example of an NDC number?

    A. 0093-0437-01
    B. 01232-543-1
    C. 9678-234-09
    D. 00781-5824-100
    E. All of the above

37. Which of the following is an example of a near miss error?

    A. A dispensing error that results in a patient taking the wrong medication.
    B. A dispensing error that results in a patient receiving another patient's prescription but realizing the error and reporting it to the pharmacy before taking any medication.
    C. An error that is caught and fixed before reaching the patient.
    D. Both B & C

38. Which FDA recall would be issued for a product that is unlikely to cause adverse health effects?

    A. Class I
    B. Class II
    C. Class III
    D. Class IV
    E. Class A

39. Which technologies can help reduce the probability of medication errors?
(Select all that apply)

    ☐ Computerized Physician Order Entry (CPOE)
    ☐ E-Prescribing
    ☐ Class A Prescription Balances
    ☐ Bar-Code Technology
    ☐ BSA Dosing

40. How many refills can a prescriber issue for a Schedule III controlled substance, and for what length of time is the prescription valid according to federal law?

    A. 12 refills, 12 months
    B. 11 refills, 12 months
    C. 5 refills, 6 months
    D. No refills, 30 days

41. Which statement best describes Concerta® (methylphenidate extended release)?

    A. A non-controlled substance used for the treatment of diarrhea.
    B. A Schedule I controlled substance with no medically accepted uses.
    C. A Schedule II controlled substance used to treat ADHD.
    D. A Schedule III controlled substance used to treat insomnia
    E. A Schedule V controlled substance used to treat opioid addiction.

42. Is the prescriber's DEA number valid on the prescription image shown below?

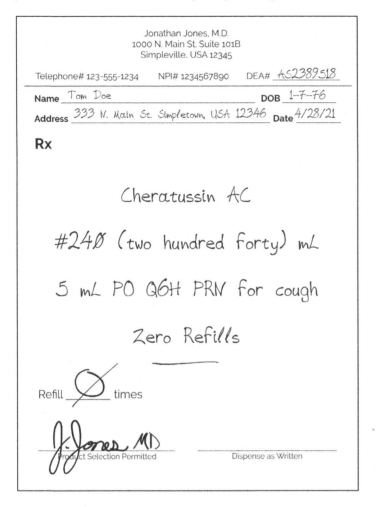

Jonathan Jones, M.D.
1000 N. Main St. Suite 101B
Simpleville, USA 12345

Telephone# 123-555-1234   NPI# 1234567890   DEA# _AS2389518_

Name _Tom Doe_   DOB _1-7-76_

Address _333 N. Main St. Simpletown, USA 12346_ Date _4/28/21_

Rx

Cheratussin AC

#240 (two hundred forty) mL

5 mL PO Q6H PRN for cough

Zero Refills

Refill ___⊘___ times

J. Jones, MD

Product Selection Permitted   Dispense as Written

A. Yes
B. No
C. Not enough information

43. How many teaspoons are equivalent to 240 mL and what is the days' supply of Cheratussin® AC for the prescription displayed in question #42?

A. 8 teaspoons/12-day supply
B. 8 teaspoons/8-day supply
C. 16 teaspoons/12-day supply
D. 48 teaspoons/12-day supply
E. 48 teaspoons/8-day supply

44. The drug prescribed in question #42 belongs to which of the following categories?

A. Non-controlled substance
B. Schedule II controlled substance
C. Schedule III controlled substance
D. Schedule V controlled substance
E. Both A & C

45. Which of the following is most useful in the event of a recall?

    A. Manufacturer address
    B. Expiration date
    C. Lot number
    D. Manufacturer phone number
    E. All of the above are equally important

46. Which of the following could be used to determine if one drug product is therapeutically equivalent to another drug product?

    A. USP Chapter <795>
    B. USP Chapter <797>
    C. The Code of Federal Regulations
    D. The Orange Book

47. Clindamycin, an antibiotic, can be used topically to treat which of the following?

    A. Acne
    B. Eczema
    C. Psoriasis
    D. Skin infections

48. If a prescriber writes a prescription for CCXL milliliters of Hydromet® oral solution, then how many milliliters should be dispensed?

    A. 8 ounces
    B. 120 mL
    C. 240 mL
    D. 360 mL
    E. 480 mL

49. According to the manufacturer, Travatan Z® eye drops should be stored at or between 2–25°C. Which environment(s) would be acceptable for storing this product?

    A. A cold environment
    B. A cool environment
    C. A room temperature environment
    D. Both B and C
    E. All of the above

50. Which of the following is used to report to the FDA an adverse event associated with a prescription drug?

    A. Compounding Record
    B. MedWatch
    C. The Federal Drug Reaction Reporting App
    D. The Drug Safety Event Recorder
    E. Medicaid

51. Which antiviral medication is used specifically for influenza?

    A. Acyclovir
    B. Ganciclovir
    C. Oseltamivir
    D. Valacyclovir

52. Which of the following describes Adipex-P® (phentermine)?

    A. Schedule IV controlled substance for weight loss
    B. Schedule V controlled substance for weight loss
    C. Non-controlled substance for ADHD
    D. Schedule V controlled substance for ADHD

53. Which antibiotic is only used for urinary tract infections?

    A. Cephalexin
    B. Ciprofloxacin
    C. Nitrofurantoin
    D. Sulfamethoxazole/Trimethoprim

54. A patient approaches the pharmacy complaining of a possible allergic reaction to a new prescription medication. Which of the following responses is most appropriate?

    A. Tell the patient to visit the emergency department
    B. Show the patient where the over the counter allergy medications are located
    C. Tell the patient to see a physician who specializes in treating allergies
    D. Tell the patient to speak to the pharmacist

55. Which antidepressant can be used for smoking cessation?

    A. Bupropion
    B. Duloxetine
    C. Nortriptyline
    D. Trazodone

56. The pharmacist wants the refrigerator temperature to be set at 6°C. What is this temperature in degrees Fahrenheit?

    A. 0°F
    B. 32°F
    C. 35°F
    D. 43°F
    E. 100°F

57. Which of the following is not a beta blocker?

    A. Albuterol
    B. Atenolol
    C. Carvedilol
    D. Metoprolol
    E. Nebivolol

58. Tanya weighs 210 pounds and has a life-threatening fungal infection. Her physician prescribes a 0.3 mg/kg dose of amphotericin B. How many micrograms of amphotericin B should Tanya receive?

    A. 29 mg
    B. 63 mg
    C. 29,000 mcg
    D. 63,000 mcg
    E. 33 mg

59. The dose of experimental drug DH671244 is 55 mg/m² every 8 hours. How many milligrams of DH671244 should be given over the course of 24 hours for a male patient that is exactly 6 feet tall and weighs 240 pounds?

    A. 190 mg
    B. 280 mg
    C. 390 mg
    D. 460 mg
    E. 530 mg

60. What is wrong with the following prescription?

Simpletown Hospital
1111 N. Main St.
Anywhere, USA 54321
Telephone# 800-555-1111
Dr. Joe Smith, MD DEA#_____

Patient Name _John Doe_____ Date _10/12/2021_

Address _222 North Main St. Sumwhere, USA 65432_____ DOB _01/07/1976_

Rx

Haloperidol 2.0 mg
Dispense #90
Take i PO QAM & ii PO QHS
2 Refills

J.S____ M.D.

_____   _____
Product Selection Permitted   Dispense as Written

    A. The insurance will not cover this medication for a 30-day supply.
    B. The prescriber used a trailing zero.
    C. The prescriber's DEA number is not written on the prescription.
    D. The prescriber did not sign on the "Dispense as Written" line.
    E. All of the above.

61. Approximately how many tablespoons are equal to 2 ounces of a liquid?

    A. 8 teaspoons
    B. 4 teaspoons
    C. 2 tablespoons
    D. 4 tablespoons
    E. ½ of a cup

62. Which of the following is not a narrow therapeutic index (NTI) drug?

    A. Carbamazepine
    B. Digoxin
    C. Losartan
    D. Phenytoin
    E. None of the above

63. Which dosage form is designed to melt at normal human body temperature?

        A. Transdermal drug delivery system
        B. Inhalation solution
        C. Ointment
        D. Suppository

64. Which medication is not used for treating depression?

        A. Venlafaxine
        B. Fluoxetine
        C. Hydralazine
        D. Mirtazapine
        E. Escitalopram

65. Which dosage form must be shaken well prior to use?

        A. Elixir
        B. Solution
        C. Suspension
        D. Cream
        E. Ointment

66. Which medication is used for the treatment of nausea and vomiting?

        A. Diflucan® (fluconazole)
        B. Imitrex® (sumatriptan)
        C. Ditropan® (oxybutynin)
        D. Zofran® (ondansetron)

67. Your pharmacy acquired 30-tablet bottles of clopidogrel 75 mg from their distributor at a WAC of $59.95. The pharmacist instructs you to set the retail price based on a markup of 12% and a dispensing fee of $11. A patient calls the pharmacy asking for the price of 60 tablets of clopidogrel 75 mg. The patient is not using insurance. Which response is correct?

        A. $78.14
        B. $145.29
        C. $156.29
        D. $176.14

68. PTCB certification must be renewed _____.

        A. Every year
        B. Every 2 years
        C. Every 3 years
        D. Every 4 years
        E. Every 5 years

69. Which dosage form should not be swallowed whole?

        A. Immediate Release Tablet
        B. Enteric Coated Tablet
        C. Extended Release Capsule
        D. Sublingual Tablet

70. Which of the following statements is correct regarding scored tablets?

    A. Scored tablets should never be split or cut.
    B. Scored tablets are designed for sublingual administration.
    C. Scored tablets always have a circular shape.
    D. Scored tablets are designed to be split easily into fractions.
    E. Scored tablets will not dissolve until they reach the small intestine.

71. Which medication can be used to treat type II diabetes?

    A. Januvia® (sitagliptin)
    B. Lopid® (gemfibrozil)
    C. Colcrys® (colchicine)
    D. Zetia® (ezetimibe)

72. Which task can be performed by a pharmacy technician?

    A. Administer immunizations
    B. Provide an over the counter drug recommendation
    C. Count and label a controlled substance prescription
    D. Provide pharmaceutical counseling

73. What is the benefit of extended release metformin (compared to immediate release metformin)?

    A. Extended release metformin is cheaper
    B. Extended release metformin has fewer gastrointestinal side effects
    C. Extended release metformin can be used for type I diabetes
    D. Extended release metformin can cause hypoglycemia

74. If the normal adult dose of clindamycin is 300 mg, then, according to Clark's Rule, what is the appropriate dose for a 4-year-old patient who weighs 60 pounds?

    A. 55 mg
    B. 100 mg
    C. 110 mg
    D. 120 mg
    E. 165 mg

75. Federal law indicates that prescription records must be kept for 2 years, but the state law where you work indicates that prescription records must be kept for 3 years. Given this information, how long should the records be kept?

    A. 2 years
    B. 2 & ½ years
    C. 3 years
    D. 4 years
    E. None of the above

76. A prescription is written for prednisone 10 mg tablets with instructions to take 4 tablets by mouth daily for 2 days, then 3 tablets daily for 2 days, then 2 tablets daily for 2 days, then 1 tablet daily for 2 days, then ½ tablet daily for 2 days, then stop. How many tablets will you need to dispense?

     A. 18 tablets
     B. 21 tablets
     C. 24 tablets
     D. 27 tablets
     E. 30 tablets

77. A prescription is written for 60 tablets of bupropion XL 150 mg with instructions for the patient to take 1 tablet by mouth once daily for 8 days and then take 2 tablets by mouth once daily thereafter. What is the correct days' supply for this prescription?

     A. 27 days
     B. 30 days
     C. 33 days
     D. 34 days
     E. 38 days

78. Approximately how long does it take for antidepressants to reach their peak effect?

     A. 60 minutes
     B. 72 hours
     C. 4 weeks
     D. 12 months

79. Which vitamin can be used to lower cholesterol and triglycerides?

     A. Vitamin A (Retinol)
     B. Vitamin B1 (Thiamine)
     C. Vitamin C (Ascorbic Acid)
     D. Vitamin B3 (Niacin)
     E. Vitamin D2 (Ergocalciferol)

80. Which insulin formulation is available without a prescription?

     A. Lantus®
     B. Novolin® 70/30
     C. Levemir®
     D. Humalog®
     E. Apidra®

81. Which product reverses the effect of warfarin?

     A. Vitamin K
     B. Aspirin
     C. Tylenol®
     D. Senna
     E. Metformin

82. Which medication is typically considered to be a high-alert medication?

    A. Citalopram
    B. Metoprolol
    C. Fluticasone
    D. Methotrexate
    E. Hydrocortisone

83. Which supplement can be used to alleviate symptoms of menopause?

    A. SAM-e
    B. Melatonin
    C. Witch Hazel
    D. Black Cohosh
    E. Red Yeast Rice

84. A 6-year-old patient needs to receive experimental drug AP22233, but there is no established pediatric dose. If the normal adult dose is 3 milligrams, what dose should the child receive according to Young's Rule?

    A. 0.33 mg
    B. 0.5 mg
    C. 0.67 mg
    D. 1 mg
    E. 1.33 mg

85. Which task cannot be performed by a pharmacy technician?

    A. Evaluate the appropriateness and safety of drug therapy
    B. Remove recalled and expired medications from stock
    C. Type prescription labels
    D. Re-stock inventory
    E. Both B & D

86. Which of the following is an example of a brand name?

    A. Albuterol HFA
    B. Lisinopril
    C. Naproxen
    D. Motrin
    E. Ibandronate

87. How many grams of each ingredient are needed to compound the prescription below?

Simpletown Hospital
1111 N. Main St.
Anywhere, USA 54321
Telephone# 800-555-1111
Dr. Joe Smith, MD DEA#_____

Patient Name John Doe   Date 10/12/2020

Address 222 North Main St. Sumwhere, USA 65432   DOB 01/07/1976

Rx

1:1 Mixture of Eucerin Cream & Triamcinolone 0.5% Ointment

Dispense 1-pound jar

AAA BID PRN for itchy rash

NR

J. Smith M.D.

_____   _____
Product Selection Permitted   Dispense as Written

A. 500 g Eucerin Cream & 500 g Triamcinolone 0.5% Ointment
B. 227 g Eucerin Cream & 227 g Triamcinolone 0.5% Ointment
C. 500 g Eucerin Cream & 500 g Triamcinolone 1% Ointment
D. 254 g Eucerin Cream & 254 g Triamcinolone 1% Ointment
E. 0.5 kg Eucerin Cream & 0.5 kg Triamcinolone 1% Ointment

88. How has Dr. Joe Smith implemented safety strategies for the bupropion prescription pictured below?

```
Simpletown Hospital
1111 N. Main St.
Anywhere, USA 54321
Telephone# 800-555-1111
Dr. Joe Smith, MD DEA#_____

Patient Name John Doe _____    Date 10/12/2020

Address 222 North Main St. Sumwhere, USA 65432      DOB 01/07/1976

Rx
                 BuPROPion XL 300 mg

                     #30 tablets

          Take one tablet by mouth once daily

                     2 Refills


J. Smith MD.

_____              _____
Product Selection Permitted             Dispense as Written
```

A. Dr. Smith used tall man lettering
B. Dr. Smith did not use any error-prone abbreviations
C. Dr. Smith did not use trailing zeros
D. All of the above

89. A patient presents a prescription for Clindamycin 300 mg capsules with instructions to take 300 mg by mouth every 6 hours for 14 days. How many capsules should you dispense?

A. 42 capsules
B. 56 capsules
C. 68 capsules
D. 72 capsules
E. Not enough information

90. What does the sig code "AU" stand for?

A. Left eye
B. Both eyes
C. Left ear
D. Both ears
E. Australia

PRACTICE EXAM
ANSWER KEY

1.   C. 143 lbs

$$65 \text{ kg } \times \frac{2.2 \text{ lb}}{\text{kg}} = 143 \text{ lb}$$

To review must-know conversion factors, see page 160.

2.   C. September 30, 2022

To review lot numbers and expiration dates, see page 204.

3.   D. Levetiracetam

BRAND NAME	GENERIC NAME
Prevacid®	Lansoprazole
Lamictal®	Lamotrigine
Atrovent®	Ipratropium
Keppra®	Levetiracetam

4.   E. Both A & C

CATEGORY	BRAND NAME	ONSET OF ACTION	DURATION OF ACTION
Rapid Acting	Apidra®, Humalog®, NovoLog®	15 - 30 min.	3 - 6 hours
Short Acting	Humulin R®, Novolin R®	30 - 60 min.	6 - 10 hours
Intermediate Acting	Humulin N®, Novolin N®	1 - 2 hours	16 - 24 hours
Long Acting	Lantus®, Levemir®, Toujeo®	1 - 2 hours	24 hours
Ultra Long Acting	Tresiba®	1 hour	24 - 40 hours

5.   B. Ophthalmic

To review the ophthalmic prostaglandin analogs, see page 64.

6.   E. Angiotensin Converting Enzyme Inhibitors

20% of patients that use an ACE inhibitor develop a dry, non-productive cough. To review ACE inhibitors, see pages 14-15.

7.   All five options should be selected.

All of the drugs listed are either NSAIDs or antibiotics. When taken with Coumadin® (warfarin), these drugs can increase the risk of bleeding. To review these drug interactions, see page 75.

8.   A. Singulair®   -   V. Montelukast
       B. Desyrel®   -   IV. Trazodone
       C. Dilantin®   -   I. Phenytoin
       D. Tessalon®   -   II. Benzonatate
       E. Valium®   -   III. Diazepam

9.   A. Meloxicam   -   III. Inflammation
       B. Fexofenadine   -   V. Allergies
       C. Olmesartan   -   IV. Hypertension
       D. Fentanyl   -   II. Pain
       E. Zolpidem   -   I. Insomnia

10. B. DEA

AGENCY	ROLE
FDA	Enforces drug manufacturing laws. Regulates prescription drug advertising and large-scale compounding
DEA	Enforces the federal Controlled Substances Act (CSA). Classifies controlled substances
OSHA	Enforces employee health and safety laws
FTC	Regulates OTC drug, medical device, cosmetic, and food advertising

11. B. Schedule II

SCHEDULE	MEDICAL USES	ABUSE POTENTIAL	DEPENDENCE POTENTIAL
C-I	No	High	High
C-II	Yes	High	High
C-III	Yes	Moderate	Moderate-Low
C-IV	Yes	Mild	Mild
C-V	Yes	Low	Low

12. B. DEA Form 222

FORM	PURPOSE
DEA Form 41	To report to the DEA the destruction of controlled substances
DEA Form 106	To report to the DEA the theft or loss of controlled substances.
DEA Form 222	To order (or to document the transfer of) Schedule I or Schedule II controlled substances

To review other DEA Forms, see page 107.

13. C. 70% isopropyl alcohol

To review pharmacy hygiene and cleaning standards, see page 130.

14. C. Vaccines

To review details regarding MedWatch and VAERS, see page 130.

15. C. iPLEDGE

REMS PROGRAM	DRUG AFFECTED
iPLEDGE	Isotretinoin*
THALIDOMID REMS	Thalidomid® (Thalidomide)
T.I.P.S.	Tikosyn® (Dofetilide)
Clozaril National Registry	Clozaril® (Clozapine)

*Multiple brand name formulations available.

16. B. 3.6 grams

An individual may purchase up to 3.6 grams of pseudoephedrine in one day, but not more than 9 grams in any 30-day period. If purchasing pseudoephedrine via mail order, the limit is 7.5 grams in any 30-day period.

17.   B. Buspirone

To review the Top 200 Drugs, see pages 66-69.

18.   D. All of the above are error-prone abbreviations

To review a list of error-prone abbreviations, see page 125.

19.   A. Mupirocin

To review the Top 200 Drugs, see pages 66-69.

20.   D. Both A & C

The DEA reclassified all hydrocodone combination products from Schedule III to Schedule II (effective October 6, 2014). According to federal law, refills are prohibited for all Schedule II controlled substances. Additionally, all prescriptions for controlled substances must include the prescriber's DEA number. There are no federal laws or rules that require any type of patient identification number to appear on the face of a prescription.

21.   B. Root-cause analysis

To review dispensing errors, see page 129.

22.   C. Hydroxyzine

To review the Top 200 Drugs, see pages 66-69.

23.   C. PO (by mouth)

"Per os" is an error-prone abbreviation because "os" could be misinterpreted as "OS" (left eye). However, "PO" is not an error-prone abbreviation. To review a list of error-prone abbreviations, see page 125.

24.   B. 2

If you know the sensitivity requirement of the balance (6 mg in this case) and the weight of a substance being measured (300 mg), you can calculate the percent error using the following equation:

$$\% \text{ Error} = \frac{\text{Sensitivity Requirement}}{\text{Measured Weight}} \times 100\% = \frac{6 \text{ mg}}{300 \text{ mg}} \times 100\% = 2\%$$

To review percent error, see pages 141-143. To memorize the common pharmacy math equations, see Appendix A on page 239.

25.   C. 36 mL

This is an alligation problem.

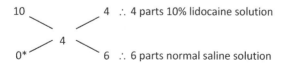

10   4 ∴ 4 parts 10% lidocaine solution

              4

0*   6 ∴ 6 parts normal saline solution

* Normal saline solution contains zero percent lidocaine.

This compound will consist of 10 parts (4 parts 10 % lidocaine solution and 6 parts normal saline solution). In other words, four-tenths (4/10) of the 90 mL prescription will be composed of the 10% lidocaine solution, and the other six-tenths (6/10) will be composed of normal saline solution (i.e., 0% lidocaine solution).

$$\frac{90 \text{ mL}}{10 \text{ parts}} \times \frac{4 \text{ parts of 10\% Lidocaine}}{1} = 36 \text{ mL of 10\% Lidocaine}$$

To review alligation alternates, see pages 155 – 158.

26.　　D. 180 tablets

To solve this problem, the first thing you must do is determine how many milligrams of allopurinol are needed to compound the entire prescription. This is a simple, one-step multiplication problem:

$$450 \text{ mL} \times \frac{40 \text{ mg}}{\text{mL}} = 18,000 \text{ mg}$$

Since we know there are 100 milligrams of allopurinol in each tablet, the next step is just as easy:

$$18,000 \text{ mg} \times \frac{\text{tablet}}{100 \text{ mg}} = 180 \text{ tablets}$$

27.　　D. Look-alike/sound-alike medications

To review look-alike/sound-alike medications, see page 122.

28.　　D. All of the above

To review Insulin and high-alert medications, see pages 40 and 123.

29.　　A. To emphasize the differences in spelling between medications with similar names.

To review tall man lettering, see page 124.

30.　　B. The use of leading zeros decreases the likelihood of an error.

To review leading zeros, see page 124.

31.　　D. Recommending an over the counter medication for a patient.

To review issues requiring pharmacist intervention, see page 128.

32.　　C. Because excessive doses can cause severe and potentially fatal bleeding.

To review high-alert medications, see page 123.

33.　　C. Pharmacist

To review issues requiring pharmacist intervention, see page 128.

34.　　D. ISMP and FDA

To review error-prone abbreviations, see page 125.

35.   C. X

A unique DEA registration number that begins with an "X" is granted to prescribers who have obtained the necessary waiver from the DEA to prescribe, administer, or dispense C-III through C-V controlled substances for the treatment of narcotic addiction outside of a narcotic treatment facility. For more on this topic, see the Drug Addiction Treatment Act section on page 108.

36.   A. 0093-0437-01

NDC numbers consist of 11 digits (a 5-digit segment to identify the manufacturer, a 4-digit segment to identify the drug product, and a 2-digit segment that is usually used to identify the package size). In some cases, when a segment contains one or more leading zeros, a leading zero will be omitted. For instance, 00093-0437-01 could be expressed in any one of the following three ways:

0093-0437-01
00093-437-01
00093-0437-1

37.   C. An error that is caught and fixed before reaching the patient.

To review near miss errors, see page 129.

38.   C. Class III

The 3 classes of FDA recalls are Class I, Class II, and Class III. The Class I recall is the most critical; in these cases, serious adverse health consequences, up to and including death, are possible. The Class III recall is the least critical; in these cases, the recalled product is unlikely to cause any adverse health consequences.

39.   The following 3 options should be selected:
- ✓ Computerized Physician Order Entry (CPOE)
- ✓ E-Prescribing
- ✓ Bar-Code Technology

Body surface area (BSA) dosing is a method of calculating therapeutic doses for certain medications (e.g., many cancer chemotherapies) based on a patient's height and weight, and the Class A prescription balance is a tool for measuring weight.

40.   C. 5 refills, 6 months

The federal Controlled Substances Act limits the number of refills on Schedule III and IV controlled substance prescriptions to a maximum of 5 refills within 6 months.

41.   C. A Schedule II controlled substance used to treat ADHD.

To review the Top 200 Drugs, see pages 66-69.

42.   B. No

When asked whether or not a DEA number is valid, you are expected to apply the 4-step process outlined on page 122. When you take the DEA number shown on the prescription (AS2389518) and apply the 4-step verification process, you see that the last digit of the DEA number should be "1;" however, the last digit of this prescriber's DEA number is "8."

43.   D. 48 teaspoons/12-day supply

This is a 2-part question. The solution to the first part involves simple unit conversion (convert milliliters to teaspoons). If you got this part wrong, go back and memorize the list of Must-Know Conversion Factors on page 200, then practice solving problems using conversion factors. The second part of this problem is a days' supply calculation (see below). If you got the wrong answer for this part, review Days' Supply Calculations on pages 170-173.

$$\frac{240 \text{ mL}}{1} \times \frac{\text{dose}}{5 \text{ mL}} \times \frac{\text{day}}{4 \text{ doses}} = 12 \text{ days}$$

44.   D. Schedule V controlled substance

A medication is categorized as either C-I, C-II, C-III, C-IV, C-V, or non-controlled. There is no way to know which schedule a medication belongs to other than memorization. To review common controlled substances, see pages 99-101.

45.   C. Lot Number

To review the topic of lot numbers, see page 204.

46.   D. The Orange Book

To review generic substitution and the Orange Book, see page 84.

47.   A. Acne

To review the Top 200 Drugs, see pages 66-69.

48.   C. 240 mL

CCXL is the Roman numeral form of the number 240. Although choice "A" (8 ounces) is equivalent to 240 mL, the question specifically asks how many **milliliters** should be dispensed. To review Roman Numerals, see pages 145-146.

49.   E. All of the above

TEMPERATURE RANGES	
Cold	2°C to 8°C (36°F to 46°F)
Cool	8°C to 15°C (46°F to 59°F)
Room Temperature	20°C to 25°C (68°F to 77°F)

All of these environments have a temperature within the range specified by the manufacturer.

50.   B. MedWatch

An adverse event associated with a prescription that was compounded should be recorded in the dispensing pharmacy's compounding record, but this would be an example of internal reporting, and the FDA would not automatically receive such a report. "The Federal Drug Reaction Reporting App," and "The Drug Safety Event Recorder" are fictitious programs (i.e., they're not real). Medicaid is a type of government-funded health insurance that provides coverage for people with limited income/resources. To review the details of MedWatch, see page 130.

51.   C. Oseltamivir

To review the Top 200 Drugs, see pages 66-69.

52.   A. Schedule IV controlled substance for weight loss

To review the Top 200 Drugs, see pages 66-69.

53.   C. Nitrofurantoin

To review the Top 200 Drugs, see pages 66-69.

54.   D. Tell the patient to speak to the pharmacist

To review issues requiring pharmacist intervention, see page 128.

55.   A. Bupropion

To review the Top 200 Drugs, see pages 66-69.

56.   D. 43°F

$$°F = \left(\frac{9}{5} \times °C\right) + 32$$

To memorize the Common Pharmacy Math Equations, see Appendix A on page 239.

57.   A. Albuterol

To review albuterol, see page 57. To review beta blockers, see page 24.

58.   C. 29,000 mcg

Pay close attention to the units. This question specifically asked for an answer in micrograms.

$$210 \text{ lb} \times \frac{\text{kg}}{2.2 \text{ lb}} \times \frac{0.3 \text{ mg}}{\text{kg}} \times \frac{1,000 \text{ mcg}}{\text{mg}} = 28,636 \text{ mcg} \therefore 29,000 \text{ mcg}$$

To review unit conversion, see page 159. To review must-know conversion factors, see page 160.

59.   C. 390 mg

The solution to this problem involves multiple steps. First, you need to calculate the patient's body surface area (BSA). To calculate BSA, you must convert height to centimeters and weight to kilograms, then enter the values into the BSA equation (see page 239). Then multiply the patient's BSA by 55 mg/m² to calculate the dose. Finally, you must multiply the dose by 3 since the patient will receive a dose every 8 hours and the question asks how many milligrams will be given in 24 hours.

60.   B. The prescriber used a trailing zero.

The use of trailing zeros could lead to interpretation errors. For example, 2 mg written as 2.0 mg could be misinterpreted as 20 mg. To review trailing zeros, see page 125.

233

61.   D. 4 tablespoons

$$\frac{2 \text{ ounces}}{1} \times \frac{30 \text{ mL}}{\text{ounce}} \times \frac{1 \text{ tablespoon}}{15 \text{ mL}} = 4 \text{ tablespoons}$$

To review unit conversion, see page 159. To review must-know conversion factors, see page 160.

62.   C. Losartan

To review narrow therapeutic index drugs, see page 84.

63.   D. Suppository

To review suppositories, see page 83.

64.   C. Hydralazine

Hydralazine is a vasodilator used for the treatment of angina.

65.   C. Suspension

To review this concept, see the illustration on page 79.

66.   D. Zofran® (ondansetron)

To review antiemetics, see page 35.

67.   B. $145.29

Retail Cost = [AWP x (1 + Markup*)] + Dispensing Fee
*Markup expressed as a decimal

Retail Cost = [($59.95/bottle x 2 bottles) x (1 + 0.12)] + $11 = $145.29

Note: A dispensing fee is charged on a per prescription basis. This fee does not increase or decrease based on the quantity dispensed.

68.   B. Every 2 years

For a summary of PTCB certification renewal requirements, see page 206.

69.   D. Sublingual Tablet

To review the details of this and other solid dosage forms, see page 80.

70.   D. Scored tablets are designed to be split easily into fractions.

To review the details of this and other solid dosage forms, see page 80.

71.   A. Januvia® (sitagliptin)

To review the Top 200 Drugs, see pages 66-69.

72.   C. Count and label a controlled substance prescription

To review the role of pharmacy technicians and issues requiring pharmacist intervention, see pages 127 and 128.

73.   B. Extended release metformin has fewer gastrointestinal side effects

To review metformin, see page 41.

74.   D. 120 mg

$$\text{Child Dose} = \frac{60 \text{ lb}}{150 \text{ lb}} \times 300 \text{ mg} = 120 \text{ mg}$$

To review Clark's Rule and other pediatric dosing equations, see pages 181-183.

75.   A. 2 years

You do not need to know specific state laws for the PTCB exam, but you should know that when federal and state laws differ, you must follow the more stringent law.

76.   B. 21 tablets

$$\left(\frac{4 \text{ tablets}}{\text{day}} \times 2 \text{ days} \right) + \left(\frac{3 \text{ tablets}}{\text{day}} \times 2 \text{ days} \right) + \left(\frac{2 \text{ tablets}}{\text{day}} \times 2 \text{ days} \right)$$

$$+ \left(\frac{1 \text{ tablet}}{\text{day}} \times 2 \text{ days} \right) + \left(\frac{0.5 \text{ tablet}}{\text{day}} \times 2 \text{ days} \right)$$

$$= 21 \text{ tablets}$$

77.   D. 34 days

After the first 8 days of therapy, the patient will have 52 tablets remaining. Those 52 tablets will be sufficient to last 26 days (52 divided by 2, since the patient takes 2 tablets daily; see math below). So, the first 8 tablets last 8 days, and the remaining 52 tablets will last 26 days. Then it is simple addition, 8 days + 26 days = 34 days.

$$\text{For the first 8 days:} \quad 8 \text{ tablets} \times \frac{\text{day}}{1 \text{ tablet}} = 8 \text{ days}$$

$$\text{After the first 8 days:} \quad 52 \text{ tablets} \times \frac{\text{day}}{2 \text{ tablets}} = 26 \text{ days}$$

78.   C. 4 weeks

To review antidepressants, see pages 36-38.

79.   D. Vitamin B3 (Niacin)

To review vitamins, see pages 72-73.

80.   B. Novolin® 70/30

Insulin Formulations Available Without a Prescription (OTC)

| Novolin® N | Novolin® R | Novolin® 70/30 |
| Humulin® N | Humulin® R | Humulin® 70/30 |

---

81.   A. Vitamin K

To review the details of the drug-nutrient interaction between warfarin and vitamin K, see page 76.

82.   D. Methotrexate

To review high-alert medications, see page 123.

83.   D. Black Cohosh

To review the Top 30 Herbal Supplements, see page 74.

84.   D. 1 mg

$$\text{Child Dose} = \frac{6}{(6 + 12)} \times 3 \text{ mg} = 1 \text{ mg}$$

To review Young's Rule and other pediatric dosing equations, see pages 181-183.

85.   A. Evaluate the appropriateness and safety of drug therapy

To review issues requiring pharmacist intervention, see page 128.

86.   D. Motrin

BRAND NAME	GENERIC NAME
ProAir®, Ventolin®, Proventil®	Albuterol HFA
Prinivil®, Zestril	Lisinopril
Aleve®, Naprosyn®	Naproxen
Motrin®, Advil®	Ibuprofen
Boniva®	Ibandronate

87.   B. 227 g Eucerin Cream & 227 g Triamcinolone 0.5% Ointment

The prescription asks for a one-pound mixture containing equal parts of Eucerin Cream and Triamcinolone 0.5% Ointment. This is a simple unit conversion problem. We already know that we need one-half pound of each ingredient. The question is: how many grams are in one-half pound? You must have the conversion factor committed to memory; there are 454 grams in 1 pound. One-half of 454 grams is 227 grams. So, to compound this prescription, you will need 227 grams of Eucerin Cream and 227 grams of Triamcinolone 0.5% Ointment. If your answer was incorrect, you need to go back to page 160 and memorize the list of Must-Know Conversion Factors.

88.   D. All of the above

To review error prevention strategies, see pages 124-126.

89.   B. 56 capsules

$$\frac{1 \text{ capsule}}{6 \text{ hours}} \times \frac{24 \text{ hours}}{\text{day}} \times \frac{14 \text{ days}}{1} = 56 \text{ capsules}$$

To review unit conversion, see page 159.

90.   D. Both ears

SIG CODE	MEANING
AD	right ear
AS	left ear
AU	both ears
OD	right eye
OS	left eye
OU	both eyes

To review more sig codes, see pages 188-191.

WANT ANOTHER PRACTICE EXAM?
WE LOVE GOING ABOVE AND BEYOND TO HELP YOU ACHIEVE YOUR GOAL OF BECOMING CERTIFIED.

THAT'S WHY WE CREATED A SECOND FULL-LENGTH PRACTICE EXAM, AVAILABLE FOR FREE AT **CPHTACADEMY.COM**

★ ★ ★ ★ CHECK IT OUT TODAY! ★ ★ ★ ★

THANK YOU!

PLEASE LEAVE A REVIEW AT AMAZON.COM

$$\% \text{ Error} = \frac{\text{Sensitivity Requirement}}{\text{Desired Weight}} \times 100\%$$

$$\text{Density} = \frac{\text{Mass (grams)}}{\text{Volume (milliliters)}}$$

$$\text{Specific Gravity} = \frac{\text{Density of Substance}}{\text{Density of Reference Substance}}$$

$$^\circ C = \frac{5}{9} \left(^\circ F - 32\right) \qquad\qquad ^\circ F = \left(\frac{9}{5} \times {^\circ C}\right) + 32$$

$$\text{BSA} = \sqrt{\frac{\text{height (cm)} \times \text{weight (kg)}}{3,600}}$$

$$\text{Child Dose (Clark's Rule)} = \frac{\text{Weight (lb)}}{150 \text{ lb}} \times \text{Adult Dose}$$

$$\text{Child Dose (Young's Rule)} = \frac{\text{Age}}{(\text{Age} + 12)} \times \text{Adult Dose}$$

$$\text{Child Dose (BSA Dosing)} = \frac{\text{BSA}}{1.73 \text{ m}^2} \times \text{Adult Dose}$$

$$\frac{\text{mg} \times \text{Valence}}{\text{Molecular Weight}} = \text{mEq} \qquad\qquad \frac{\text{mEq} \times \text{Molecular Weight}}{\text{Valence}} = \text{mg}$$

$$\text{Retail Cost} = [\text{AWP} \times (1 + \text{Markup*})] + \text{Dispensing Fee}$$
*Markup expressed as a decimal

THE $20 GUARANTEE

If you purchased a brand-new copy of *PTCB Exam Simplified 4th Edition*, claimed (and used) the free bonus content (see page 1), and subsequently failed the exam, then send an email with "GUARANTEE" in the subject line to **guarantee@rxstudyguides.com** and include the information outlined below.

1. Your full name and mailing address.
2. The date you sent the email requesting the free bonus content.
3. Proof of purchase (e.g., a screenshot of the receipt showing you bought the book new).
4. A picture of your official PTCB exam results showing that you failed.

EXCEPTIONS

Please note that customers who purchased the book in "used" condition are **not** eligible for this guarantee. Furthermore, this guarantee is **invalid** if a more up-to-date version/edition of *PTCB Exam Simplified* was available when the customer purchased the book.

If you're eligible for the guarantee, we'll issue a $20 credit in the form of an Amazon gift card.

Thank you!
David A Heckman, PharmD

Made in the USA
Monee, IL
06 May 2022

95985651R00136